ESSENTIAL EMERGENCY PROCEDURAL SEDATION AND PAIN MANAGEMENT

EDITOR

Rahim Valani, MD, CCI

Assistant Professor of Medicine and
McMaster University
Canada

SERIES EDITOR

Kaushal H. Shah, MD

Associate Professor
Mt. Sinai School of Medicine
New York, New York

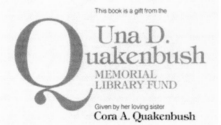

Senior Acquisitions Editor: Frances DeStefano
Product Director: Julia Seto
Production Manager: Alicia Jackson
Senior Manufacturing Manager: Benjamin Rivera
Senior Marketing Manager: Angela Panetta
Design Coordinator: Holly McLaughlin
Production Service: Aptara, Inc.

Library of Congress Cataloging-in-Publication Data

Essential emergency procedural sedation and pain management / editor, Rahim Valani.
     p. ; cm. – (Essential emergency medicine series)
  Includes bibliographical references.
  ISBN 978-1-4511-1606-9
  I. Valani, Rahim. II. Series: Essential emergency medicine series.
  [DNLM: 1. Analgesia–methods–Handbooks. 2. Conscious Sedation–methods–Handbooks.
3. Anesthetics, Combined–Handbooks. 4. Emergency Service, Hospital–Handbooks.
5. Pain–therapy–Handbooks. WO 39]
  LC classification not assigned
  617.9′6–dc23
                                                                                          2011030137

RRS1108

Dedication

To my parents and brothers for their support and inspiration over the years, and supporting my ideas; my teachers, mentors, and colleagues who have taught me the ropes of being a physician and an educator; my friends for their understanding and support.

In memory of my father who was a scholar in his own right. His integrity and compassion have made me who I am.

Contributors

Tracy-Lynn Akitt, BA, CLSt.Dipl., CLS
Child Life Specialist
Emergency Department
McMaster Children's Hospital
Hamilton, Ontario, Canada

Sadie Bartram, BASc, CCLS
Child Life Specialist
Emergency Department
McMaster Children's Hospital
Hamilton, Ontario, Canada

Sheryl Christie, BA, MA, CCLS
Certified Child Life Specialist
McMaster Children's Hospital
Hamilton, Ontario, Canada

Leanne Drehmer, BSc, BScPhm, RPh
Clinical Pharmacist
Emergency Department
McMaster Children's Hospital
Hamilton, Ontario, Canada

Mark Freedman, MD, FRCPC
Lecturer
Sunnybrook Health Sciences Centre
University of Toronto
Toronto, Ontario, Canada

Jeff Gadsden, MD, FRCPC, FANZCA
Assistant Professor of Clinical Anesthesiology
Columbia University College of Physicians &
   Surgeons
Director of Regional Anesthesia
Anesthesiology Department
St. Luke's-Roosevelt Hospital Center
New York, New York

Jeffrey Glassberg, MD, MA
Instructor
Emergency Medicine
Mount Sinai School of Medicine
New York, New York

Jessica Hernandez, MD
Department of Emergency Medicine
St. Luke's-Roosevelt Hospital Center, Columbia
   University College of Physicians and
   Surgeons
New York, New York

Tomislav Jelic, MD
Department of Emergency Medicine
University of Manitoba
Winnipeg, Manitoba, Canada

Christian LaRiviere, MD, FRCPC-EM
Lecturer
Department of Emergency Medicine
University of Manitoba
Winnipeg, Manitoba, Canada

Jarone Lee, MD, MPH
Department of Critical Care
Massachusetts General Hospital
Harvard Medical School
Boston, Massachusetts

Brian Levy, MD
Division of Emergency Medicine
McMaster University
Hamilton, Ontario, Canada

Sean Moore, MD, CMn FACEP, FRCPC
Assistant Professor
Department of Emergency Medicine
University of Ottawa
Ottawa, Ontario, Canada

David Ng, MD, CCFP-EM
Lecturer
University Health Network
University of Toronto
Toronto, Ontario, Canada

Karen E. Paling, BA, CLSt Dipl., CCLS
Certified Child Life Specialist
McMaster Children's Hospital
Hamilton, Ontario, Canada

Elaine Rabin, MD
Assistant Professor
Department of Emergency Medicine
Mount Sinai School of Medicine
New York, New York

**Sharon Ramagnano, RN, BScN,
MSN/MHA, ENC©**
Advanced Practice Nurse ED
Emergency/Trauma Department
Sunnybrook Health Sciences Centre
Toronto, Ontario, Canada

Savithri Ratnapalan, MBBS, Med
Associate Professor
Division of Paediatric Emergency Medicine and
    Pharmacology/Toxicology
The Hospital for Sick Children
Toronto, Ontario, Canada

Suzan Schneeweiss, MD, Med, FRCPC
Associate Professor
Division of Paediatric Emergency Medicine
The Hospital for Sick Children
Toronto, Ontario, Canada

Hareishun Shanmuganathan, MBBS
Department of Emergency Medicine
University of Manitoba
Winnipeg, Manitoba, Canada

Jonathan Sherbino, MD, Med, FRCPC
Assistant Professor
McMaster University
Hamilton, Ontario, Canada

Patricia Shi, MD
Assistant Professor
Hematology-Oncology Director
Adult Sickle Cell Program
The Mount Sinai School of Medicine
New York, New York

Greg Soto, ACP, BA, Bed
Paramedic Educator
Hamilton Health Sciences Centre for
    Paramedic Education & Research
Hamilton, Ontario, Canada

Alexadra Stefan, MD, MSc, FRCPC
Sunnybrook Health Sciences Centre
University of Toronto
Toronto, Ontario, Canada

Angela Stone, MSc, MD, FRCPC
Emergency Medicine and Critical Care
    Physician
Sunnybrook Health Sciences Centre
Toronto, Ontario, Canada

Vince Teo, BScPhm, PharmD
Clinical Pharmacist
Department of Emergency Services
Sunnybrook Health Sciences Centre
Toronto, Ontario, Canada

**Rahim Valani, MD, CCFP-EM, FRCPC, M.
Med. Ed**
Assistant Professor of Medicine
    and Pediatrics
McMaster University
Hamilton, Ontario, Canada

**Michelle Welsford, Bsc, MD, ABEM, FACEP,
FRCPC**
Associate Professor
McMaster University
Medical Director
Hamilton Health Sciences Centre for
    Paramedic Education & Research
Hamilton Health Sciences
Hamilton, Ontario, Canada

Nelson Wong, MD
Department of Emergency Medicine
Mount Sinai Medical Centre
New York, New York

Andrew Woorster, MD, MSc
Associate Professor
Division of Emergency Medicine
McMaster University
Hamilton, Ontario, Canada

Shelly Zubert, FRCPC, BSc, BA
Department of Emergency Medicine and
 Critical Care
University of Manitoba
Winnipeg, Manitoba, Canada

Preface

Procedural Sedation and Analgesia (PSA) is commonly utilized in the Emergency Department (ED) for patients undergoing painful procedures. It is now an essential interprofessional skill required in the ED for effective and timely patient management.

This handbook is designed to provide the reader with a guide on the subject of procedural sedation and analgesia. With increasing competencies required by emergency room clinicians, the need for an organized approach to PSA that is consistent with best practices is essential.

This book is divided into three sections. The first part deals with procedural sedation. A step-by-step approach to PSA is outlined along with medications commonly used. The second part deals with pain management and regional anesthesia. It is important for the clinician to understand the importance of treating pain and the best modalities. The final section deals with a systems based approach to pain management using current evidence. Also in the text are special chapters dedicated to pediatric care and chronic pain which are not well described in general emergency medicine texts.

The simple format of the book makes it easy to read and access information quickly.

Acknowledgments

I would like to express my appreciation to several people who have made this book possible. To all the contributing chapter authors for their time in helping to put this book together in addition to their already demanding jobs. To my colleagues at McMaster Hamilton Health Sciences Centre and Toronto East General Hospital, I am grateful for their patience as I continued to work on completing this book. To Kaushal Shah for his advice and guidance as the series editor. My thanks to the folks at Lippincott Williams & Wilkins, including Fran DeStefano, Julia Seto, and Samir Roy at Aptara, for their guidance and review process. Also, a special thanks to George Barille for the excellent illustrations.

Contents

Procedural Sedation

Introduction to Procedural Sedation

Rahim Valani

Procedural Sedation and Analgesia

- Procedural sedation is the technique of administering a sedative or dissociative agent to induce a state that allows the patient to tolerate unpleasant procedures.
- Also known as procedural sedation and analgesia (PSA) if analgesia is administered concomitantly.
- Now advocated as a core competency in emergency medicine.
- Sedation is a continuum (see Figure 1.1 and Table 1.1):

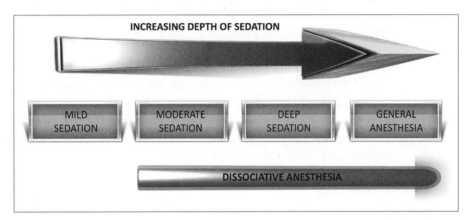

FIGURE 1.1: Sedation is a continuum, and a patient can easily move from deep sedation to general anesthesia.

- PSA is a common practice in the emergency department (ED). The goals of PSA are as follow:
  - Provide the patient with a safe environment where a painful or unpleasant procedure is required.
  - Alleviate patient anxiety.
  - Minimize physical discomfort.
  - Maximize amnesia.
  - Control motor behavior and movement if necessary so as to perform painful/ unpleasant procedures such as a lumbar puncture or fracture reduction.
  - Minimize the risk of the procedure, and ensure safe discharge of the patient from the ED.

TABLE 1.1: Continuum of sedation: levels of sedation and analgesia

	Responsiveness	Airway	Ventilation	Cardiovascular function
Mild sedation (anxiolysis)	Responds to verbal commands	Unaffected	Unaffected	Unaffected
Moderate sedation	Purposeful response to verbal or tactile stimuli	No intervention required	Adequate	Usually maintained
Deep sedation	Purposeful response to painful stimuli	Intervention may be required	May be inadequate	Usually maintained
General anesthesia	Unarousable	Intervention required	Inadequate	Impaired

- Appropriate policies and protocols enable a safe practice within the ED.
  - Ensure quality control while minimizing risks and adverse outcomes.
  - Preprinted orders and monitoring sheets should be a requirement for any department performing PSA.
- There is an increased need for the use of PSA in the ED due to the following:
  - Hospital overcrowding – there may be a potential to avoid an admission to the hospital by performing the procedure in the ED and discharging the patient home safely.
  - Limited availability of anesthesia – the anesthesia team may be in the operating room, and not available for PSA either in the ED or in the operating room.
  - Increased training of emergency physicians in PSA.
- The most common procedures using PSA performed in the ED are as follow:
  - Orthopedic procedures (most common, and includes dislocations, fracture reductions, and immobilization/splinting).
  - Abscess incision and drainage.
  - Laceration repair.
  - Cardioversion.
  - Foreign body removal.
  - Lumbar puncture.
  - Endoscopy.
- The role of PSA is expanding in the ED as it has been shown to:
  - Increase convenience of the patient – they no longer need to wait to go to the operating room.
  - Accessibility – procedures can now be done in the ED so as to facilitate easier access.
  - Cost-effectiveness by reducing wait times, earlier patient discharge, and avoidance of operating room personnel and time.
- Exclusion criteria and contraindications for ED sedation include:
  - Sedation time >30 minutes.
  - Patient with a potentially difficult airway (see Chapter 2).

- Patient with ASA functional class III or greater (see Table 4.2).
- Patients who are hemodynamically unstable.
- A patient who is known to be intubated shortly for another procedure/surgery.
- Lack of personnel experienced in airway management, advanced life support, and unfamiliarity with medications.
- Lack of appropriate monitoring equipment.
- Patient has a known allergy or sensitivity to the choice of drugs.

- Complication rate of PSA estimated to be <1 percent in the hospitals and specialties routinely practicing PSA.
  - Adverse event rate is estimated at 2–3% in pediatric patients.
  - The most common complication is respiratory depression and airway obstruction.
  - Medication error is another common cause.
    - Prescription error rate if 5.5 per 1,000 ED medication orders written.
    - The majority are due to dosing errors. Others are due to similar packaging of drugs, illegible orders, and drug interactions.
- Many of the complications related to PSA can be prevented by the following:
  - Appropriate monitoring and recognition of respiratory depression or arrest.
  - Adequate monitoring.
  - Ensuring the correct dose of medications (avoid drug calculation error).
  - Careful titration of medications.
  - Appropriate patient assessment.
  - Avoiding drug–drug interactions.
  - Personnel present who are trained in airway management and resuscitation.

Steps for Procedural Sedation and Analgesia (See Chapter 4)

Preparation

- Determine the need for the procedure, and also the following:
  - Availability of space and personnel in the department to safely conduct the procedure and sedation.
  - Sedation should take place in a central, well-maintained area of the ED that has capabilities for resuscitation and airway management.
- Provide the patient with appropriate information regarding the procedure, the need for sedation (informed consent should include benefits, risks, and limitations of therapy), anticipated changes, and expected duration of PSA.
  - Written or verbal consent should be documented.
- Prepare necessary equipment for monitoring (see Chapter 6).

Personnel

- Appropriate personnel trained in PSA and resuscitation must be present.
- Require personnel for the following:
  - Monitoring of patient.

- Physician responsible for medications used during PSA and airway management (can also use respiratory therapists for airway management).
- Person who will actually perform the procedure (different from the one giving the medications).
- Additional personnel/assistants as required.

Patient Assessment (See Chapters 5 and 6)

- Want to ensure a thorough history and physical examination.
- Pay particular attention to ASA functional status (see Table 4.2), airway assessment, and other anticipated complications.
- Assess the risk of conducting the procedural sedation in the ED versus the need to take the patient to the operating room.

Equipment and Presedation Interventions (See Chapters 2, 3, and 6)

- Medications and reversal agents drawn and ready at the bedside.
- Airway equipment, including oral airways, bag-valve mask ventilation, and intubation equipment prepared.
- Patient with full cardiorespiratory monitoring (see Chapter 6).

Procedural Sedation and Analgesia (See Chapter 5)

- See Chapter 3 on pharmacology of procedural sedation.
- The patient must be monitored continuously with objective physiological monitors and qualitative clinical assessment.
- Patient needs appropriate monitoring, including:
  - Continuous cardiac monitoring.
  - Pulse oximetry.
  - Capnography.
  - Properly trained support should continuously monitor the patient and an appropriately trained emergency physician or other credentialed specialist (like a respiratory therapist) should be present.
- The choice of the agent depends on various factors:
  - Experience of practitioner.
  - Preference of practitioner.
  - Requirements imposed by the procedure.
  - The likelihood of producing a deeper level of sedation than anticipated.

Postsedation Recovery (See Chapter 5)

- Ensure that the patient is fully awake and alert for safe discharge from the ED.
- Printed instructions for family members/caregivers.

Summary

- PSA is an important skill for emergency physicians.
- Appropriate personnel with the necessary skill set are necessary for safe practice in the ED.

Suggested Reading

American Academy of Pediatrics. Guidelines for monitoring and management of pediatric patients during and after sedation for diagnostic and therapeutic procedures: an update. Pediatrics 2006;118:2587–2606.

American College of Emergency Physicians. Clinical policy: procedural sedation and analgesia in the emergency department. Ann Emerg Med 2005;45:177–196.

American Society of Anesthesiologists. Practice guidelines for sedation and analgesia by non-anesthesiologists. Anesthesiology 2002;96:1004–1017.

Bahn EL, Holt KR. Procedural sedation and analgesia: a review of new concepts. Emerg Med Clin N Am 2005;23:503–517.

Brown TB, Lovato LM, Parker D. Procedural sedation in the acute care setting. Am Fam Physician 2005;71:85–90.

Crystal CS, McArthur TJ, Harrison B. Anesthetic and procedural sedation techniques for wound management. Emerg Med Clin N Am 2007;25:41–71.

Green SM. Research advances in procedural sedation and analgesia. Ann Emerg Med 2007;49:31–36.

Innes G, Murphy M, Nijssen-Jordan C, et al. Procedural sedation and analgesia in the emergency department: Canadian consensus guidelines. J Emerg Med 1999;17:145–156.

Kaplan RF, Yang CI. Sedation and analgesia in pediatric patients for procedures outside the operating room. Anesthesiol Clin North America 2002;20:181–194.

Miller MA, Levy P, Patel M. Procedural sedation and analgesia in the emergency department: what are the risks? Emerg Med Clin N Am 2005;23:551–572.

Miner J, Burton J. Clinical practice advisory: emergency department procedural sedation with propofol. Ann Emerg Med 2007;50:182–187.

Smally AJ, Nowicki TA. Sedation in the emergency department. Curr Opin Anaesthesiol 2007;20:379–383.

2 Airway Assessment and Management for Procedural Sedation

Angela Stone and Mark Freedman

Introduction

- Ensuring adequate patient ventilation and oxygenation during procedural sedation is essential.
  - Most common adverse event during procedural sedation is respiratory depression.
  - Appropriate assessment involves recognizing challenges in airway management and preparing for respiratory depression and apnea.
- Procedural sedation requires a dedicated physician and nurse skilled in airway management and knowledgeable about potential complications.

Airway Assessment

- Assessment of the patient's airway is essential to anticipate challenges and complications to managing potential respiratory depression (see Figure 2.1).
- The goal of airway evaluation is to identify characteristics that may predispose a patient to airway obstruction, difficult bag-valve mask (BVM) ventilation, or a difficult intubation.
- Predicting these challenges will allow preparing for appropriate airway adjuncts and tailor clinical observation.

Patient History

- A brief assessment of the patient's medical history may alert you to conditions that may predispose to challenges in airway management:
  - History of difficult intubations in the past.
  - Modified oral or airway anatomy (genetic or prior surgery).
  - History of airway problems (e.g., reactive airway disease and sleep apnea).

Physical Examination

- A thorough physical examination is necessary to adequately assess a patient's airway.
- The patient should be observed and examined and the following documented in the airway assessment:
  - Look (front and side profile, in mouth).

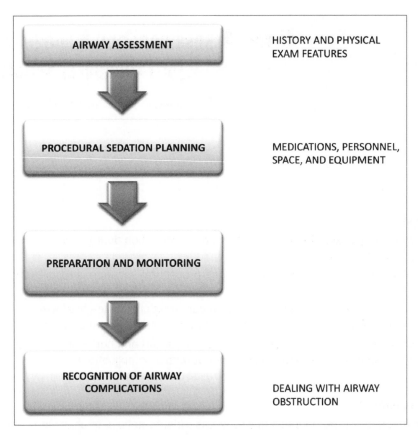

FIGURE 2.1: Overview of airway assessment and management during procedural sedation.

- Teeth (prominent incisors, crowns, dentures, loose or chipped teeth).
  - Cervical spine mobility.
- Have the patient flex and extend the head and neck.
  - Mouth Opening.
- Have the patients open their mouth as wide as possible.
- The patient should be able to insert three fingers between the incisors ideally.
  - Size of the mandible is equal to hyomental distance and thyromental distance.
    - During laryngoscopy, the tongue is pushed into the mandibular space by the blade.
      - If the mandible is too small, there will be insufficient room for the tongue to be displaced forward while the posterior tongue and epiglottis will obstruct the view of the glottis.
    - Hyomental distance – distance from hyoid bone to mentum (chin).
      - Three fingerbreadths of the patient is equal to adequate distance.
    - Thyromental distance – distance from the thyroid cartilage (Adam's apple) to the undersurface of the mandible.
      - Two fingerbreadths of the patient is equal to adequate distance.

- Oral Access
  - ▶ The size of tongue in relation to the oral cavity is assessed using the Mallampati classification.

Mallampati Classification
- The patient should be examined sitting with the head of the bed in a neutral position, the mouth opened as wide as possible, and the tongue protruded maximally.
- Visibility of the oral and pharyngeal structures (i.e., uvula, tonsillar pillars, and soft palate) are used to predict difficulty with ventilation and intubation.
  - For example, Class IV (hard palate visible only) suggests potentially difficult ventilation and intubation (Figure 2.2).

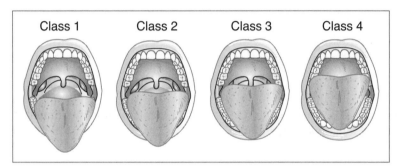

FIGURE 2.2: Airway assessment using the Mallampati classification.

Predicting Upper Airway Obstruction and Difficult Ventilation
- Predictors of difficult BVM ventilation include:
  - Beard and facial hear.
  - Obesity (BMI >26).
  - Older patients (age >55 years).
  - Edentulous.
  - History of obstructive sleep apnea.
- Two or more of the above has a 72% specificity and 73% sensitivity for difficult BVM ventilation.

Preparation and Monitoring
- Appropriate monitoring during procedural sedation is crucial, and should include the following:
  - Pulse oximetry.
  - Capnography.
  - Clinical observation.
- See Chapter 6 on monitoring during PSA.

Recognition of Airway Complications

Causes of Airway Obstruction

- Airway compromise from obstruction can occur at any level of the oropharyngeal–tracheobronchial passage.
    - Upper airway.
- Tongue (due to decreased level of consciousness causing tongue to displace posteriorly or modified anatomy).
- Soft-tissue swelling.
- Blood or vomitus.
- Direct injury.
    - Larynx.
- Foreign material.
- Soft-tissue swelling.
- Direct injury.
    - Lower airway.
- Secretions, edema, blood.
- Bronchospasm.
- Aspiration of gastric contents.
- Propfol and ketamine can be used simultaneously yet from separate syringes thus allowing their independent titration.

Recognizing Airway Obstruction

- Look for:
    - Chest/abdominal movement during sedation.
    - Condensation in the face mask.
- Listen at mouth and nose for breath sounds and abnormal sounds (gurgling, stridor, wheezing).
- Abnormal sounds due to airway obstruction:
    - Snoring – obstruction of upper airway by tongue.
    - Gurgling – obstruction of the upper airway with blood, secretions, vomit, etc.
    - Wheezing – narrowing of the lower airways/bronchospasm.
    - Silence – complete airway obstruction (i.e., laryngospasm).
- Feel at mouth and nose for expired air.

Airway Management

- BVM ventilation is a skill that is typically easy to perform. All personnel who are performing PSA need to have this skill.
- When challenges occur, the best response is that of a staged response, rather than immediately resorting to advanced airway placement.
- The vast majority of the time, noninvasive measures to treat airway obstruction (i.e., repositioning, airway adjuncts, BVM techniques) is all that is needed, and advanced airway placement can be avoided.

- In the event that advanced airway placement fails, knowing methods to trouble shoot difficulties with BVM ventilation is essential.
  - A combination of repositioning, placing an oral airway, and two-handed technique focusing on good jaw thrust is almost always successful.
  - These techniques focus on preventing the tongue from obstructing the upper airway.

Maneuvers to Open the Airway
- Head tilt, chin lift.
  - This maneuver is used to anatomically "open" the airway or place the patient in a sniffing position.
- Jaw thrust.
  - Inability to ventilate due to airway obstruction is often times corrected by using the chin-lift, jaw-thrust maneuver.
  - Ensure that the correct size face mask for a BVM is placed on the patient and held in place.
  - The mandible is elevated so as to pull forward the connecting soft tissues/tongue to relieve the obstruction.

Bag-Valve Mask Ventilation
- Knowing how to effectively ventilate a patient using a BVM (i.e., AmbuBag, Laerdal Bag) is a life-saving skill.
- Effective ventilation depends on good positioning, maneuvers that open the patient's airway, and using adjuncts to overcome airway obstruction.

Oral and Nasal Airways
- Oral and nasal airways are useful adjuncts to airway management in patients who are in moderate to deep sedation and are difficult to ventilate.
  - They act to open the airway in patients who are prone to obstruction due to body habitus or deep sedation.
  - Avoid pushing in or forcing an oral airway in a patient who is gagging.

Oral Airways
- Not tolerated in awake or mildly sedated patients.
- Appropriate size is by measuring from the front teeth of the patient to the angle of the mandible.

Nasal Airways
- Better tolerance in awake, mildly sedated patients than oral airways.
- The length of the airway is measured from the nares to the tragus of the ear.
- It should be lubricated and placed by advancing the airway straight back and close to the medial wall of the nares.
- Exercise caution in those patients who may be on anticoagulants as bleeding may occur.

Advanced Airway Techniques

Laryngeal Mask Airway

- The laryngeal mask airway (LMA) is an ovoid silicone mask with an inflatable rim that is inserted blindly into the pharynx.
- Its advantages are the following:
  - Ease of use.
  - Extremely high success rate with little training.
  - Low complication rate.
- Works as a potential alternative to endotracheal intubation when personnel are inexperienced or as a temporizing role.

Endotracheal Intubation

- If appropriate patient history, physical examination, planning, and use of noninvasive airway management skills are performed, intubation should not be necessary during PSA.
- The decision to intubate should be based on three essential criteria:
  - Failure to maintain or protect airway.
  - Failure to oxygenate or ventilate.
  - Anticipate the need for intubation.

Summary

- Having the essential skills for airway management is necessary for PSA in the emergency department.
- Appropriate planning and selection of patients can avoid potential airway complications.

Suggested Reading

Deitch, et al. The utility of supplemental oxygen during emergency department procedural sedation and analgesia with midazolam and fentanyl: a randomized controlled trial. Ann Emerg Med 2007;49(1):1–8.

Godwin, et al. Clinical policy: procedural sedation and analgesia in the emergency department. Ann Emerg Med 2005;45:177–196.

Green SM. Research advances in procedural sedation and analgesia. Ann Emerg Med 2007;49(1):31–36.

Jubran A. Pulse oximetry. In: Tobin MJ, ed. Principles and practice of intensive care monitoring. New York: McGraw Hill, 1998.

Kovacs G, Law AJ. Airway management in emergencies. New York; McGraw-Hill, 2008.

Krauss et al. Capnography for procedural sedation and analgesia in the emergency department. Ann Emerg Med 2007;50(2):172–181.

Langeron O, et al. Prediction of difficult mask ventilation. Anesthesiology 2000;92:1229–1236.

Marx, et al. Rosen's emergency medicine: concepts & clinical practice, 6th ed. St. Louis, MO: Mosby, 2006.

McFadyen JG. Respiratory gas analysis in theatre: capnography. Anaesthesia 2000;11(7):1–2.

Walker. Is capnography necessary for propofol sedation? Ann Emerg Med. 2004;44(5):549–550.

3   Pharmacology of Procedural Sedation

Vince Teo

Choosing Medications for PSA

- Procedural sedation has relied on a variety of pharmacological agents for the following:
    - Give sedation (sedatives).
    - Relieve pain (analgesics).
    - Cause a dissociative state (dissociative agents).
- These agents, either alone or used in combination allow the patient to better tolerate any pain or discomfort associated with the procedure.
- The ideal pharmacological agent for procedural sedation is able to produce:
    - Optimal sedation and analgesia rapidly.
    - Has a short duration of action to facilitate a quick recovery without recollection of procedure.
    - Does not cause any adverse events (such as respiratory depression).
- Current classes of medication employed include:
    - Benzodiazepines (e.g., midazolam).
    - Opioids (e.g., fentanyl and morphine).
    - Propofol.
    - Etomidate.
    - Ketamine.

Agents for Use in Procedural Sedation (Table 3.1)

Midazolam

- Benzodiazepines promote the binding of the inhibitory neurotransmitter, gamma-aminobutyric acid (GABA) to GABA receptors, enhancing their activity.
- Midazolam is similar to other benzodiazepines exhibiting the following properties:
    - Sedation.
    - Amnesia.
    - Anxiolysis.
    - Anticonvulsant.
    - Muscle relaxant.
- It has a rapid onset and short duration of action without active metabolites.

TABLE 3.1: Medications used for procedural sedation

Drug	Dose		Onset	Duration	Contraindications
Midazolam	Initial: 0.02–0.1 mg/kg (max 2.5 mg [1.5 mg in elderly]) Repeat 25% of dose q 3 min Cumulative max 5 mg (3.5 mg in elderly)	Inject slowly over 2 min (use 1 mg/mL)	1–2 min	30–60 min	
Propofol	Initial 0.5–1 mg/kg IV May repeat 0.5 mg/kg increments q 3–5 min	Shake well Inject slowly over 3–5 min	<1 min	3–10 min	Allergy to soybean or egg products Hypersensitivity to EDTA or sodium metabisulfite
Etomidate	0.2 mg/kg	Over 30–60 sec	<1 min	3–5 min (full recovery 5–15 min)	
Ketamine	IV 1–2 mg/kg Then 0.25–0.5 mg/kg q 5–10 min		1 min	15–10 min	HTN Increased ICP Psychosis
Fentanyl	1–1.5 mcg/kg IV titrate 1 mcg/kg q 3 min		1–2 min	30–60 min	
Atropine	0.5–1 mg q 5 min (bradycardia) 0.4–0.6 mg (salivation or secretions)	Rapid IV push	Rapid		Closed angle glaucoma Tachycardia Obstructive GI disease or ileus Myasthenia gravis
Naloxone	0.1–0.2 mg IV		1 min IV 10–15 min IM	15–30 min	
Flumazenil	0.1–0.2 mg IV may repeat in 1 min	Infuse over 15 sec Cumulative max 0.05 mg/kg (or 1 mg)	<1 min	45 min	

Indication/Properties

Sedation	Amnesia	Anxiolysis	Analgesia	Dissociation	Pros	Cons	Other
✓	✓	✓			Longer safety record/ experience with use Anticonvulsant properties	Requires 2nd agent for analgesia Hypotension Respiratory depression	
✓	✓				Rapid onset + recovery Anticonvulsant and anti-emetic properties	CV depression Hypotension can cause rapidly deepening sedation	No analgesic properties
✓	✓				No histamine release Minimal CV, respiratory effects	Myoclonus Injection site pain Transiently lowers cerebral blood flow (slight to moderate ↓ ICP usually just several minutes)	No analgesic properties
			✓	✓	Safety data in paeds	Emergence delirium (especially adults) Myoclonus Laryngospasm; Hypersecretions Agitation Nystagmus CV stimulation	
			✓		Minimal CV depression; reversible Proven safety	Requires 2nd agent for sedation Repeat dose usually required Cough Hiccups Vomiting Itchiness	
							May be given as pretreatment to prevent excessive salivation with ketamine
						Very safe	Not routine
						Can cause seizures Benzodiazepine withdrawal	Not routine

- Dosing:
  - Initial 0.02–0.1 mg/kg (maximum 2.5 mg [1.5 mg elderly]).
  - May repeat 25% of dose every 3 minutes (maximum of 5 mg cumulative dose [3.5 mg elderly]).
- Availability and administration:
  - 1 mg/mL – 10 mL vial containing 10 mg.
  - 5 mg/mL – 1 mL vial containing 5 mg.
  - Direct Injection IV slowly over 2 minutes (1 mg/mL concentration should be used to help facilitate this).
- Onset:
  - 1–2 minutes.
- Duration:
  - 30–60 minutes.
- Pharmacokinetics:
  - Midazolam has a rapid onset and short duration of action without active metabolites.
  - It is highly lipophilic, resulting in a relatively large volume of distribution (compared to other benzodiazepines).
    - ▶ Thus, its half-life increases significantly in obese patients.
  - It is metabolized in the liver, a substrate of the CYP3A4 isoenzyme, and is excreted primarily in the urine.
- Contraindications:
  - Hypersensitivity to midazolam or any component of the formulation (benzyl alcohol).
- Adverse effects:
  - Respiratory depression (dose and infusion rate dependent).
  - Apnea (dose and infusion rate dependent).
  - Hypotension.
  - Deep sedation.
  - Impaired coordination.
  - Diminished reflexes.
- Monitoring:
  - See Chapter 6 on monitoring during procedural sedation.
- Special considerations and pearls:
  - Wait at least 2 minutes to assess response before administering subsequent doses.
  - Midazolam does NOT have any analgesic properties.
    - ▶ For painful procedures, consider second agent for analgesia.
  - Patients premedicated with an opioid (e.g., fentanyl) should have dosages reduced by ~25%.
  - Co-administration with other CNS depressants (benzodiazepines, barbiturates, opioids, other sedatives) will increase sedation and the risk of respiratory depression.

- Concomitant use of CYP3A4 inhibitors (e.g., azole antifungals, erythromycin, clarithromycin, verapamil, propofol) may increase levels of midazolam.
- Patients with hepatic dysfunction or severe CHF may have experienced prolonged effects.
- When used in combination with fentanyl, respiratory depression may occur in up to 25% of patients.

Propofol
- Propofol is an ultra-short-acting non-opioid, non-barbiturate sedative-hypnotic agent.
- Its exact mechanism of action is unknown, but it is thought to enhance the binding of GABA to its receptor sites.
- It has sedative, amnestic, anticonvulsant, and anti-emetic properties.
- It does not have analgesic properties.
- Main benefits are that it has a quick onset and short duration of action resulting in a rapid recovery.
    - However, due to its potency, there is a risk to the patient of quickly progressing to deep sedation.
- Dosing:
    - Loading dose: 0.5–1 mg/kg IV.
    - May repeat 0.5 mg/kg IV every 3–5 minutes.
- Availability and administration:
    - 10 mg/mL – 20 mL, 50 mL, 100 mL vials available.
    - Propofol is available as an emulsion. Shake well prior to use.
    - Inject IV slowly over 3–5 minutes.
- Onset:
    - <1 minute.
- Duration of action:
    - 5–10 minutes (full recovery within 10–15 min).
- Pharmacokinetics:
    - Propofol is available in a soybean oil emulsion.
    - Although it achieves therapeutic concentrations in the CNS rapidly, it is rapidly redistributed to muscle and fat tissue, resulting in an effective duration of action (~10 min) much shorter than its half-life (15–45 hr).
- Contraindications:
    - Hypersensitivity to soybean oil or egg products. (Emulsifier in the formulation is derived from egg).
    - Hypersensitivity to EDTA or sodium metabisulfite (preparations of propofol contain either one of these agents as a preservative).
- Adverse effects:
    - Hypotension (may occur in up to 30% of patients).
    - Bradycardia.
    - Respiratory depression/apnea (up to 25%).
    - Site injection pain (15–20%).

- A rapid deepening of sedation.
- Spontaneous musculoskeletal movements (twitching, jerking or hands, arms, feet and legs) (3–10%).
- Monitoring:
  - See Chapter 6 on monitoring during procedural sedation.
- Special considerations:
  - Strict aseptic technique is important when preparing and administering propofol since the lipid vehicle is capable of supporting bacterial growth.
  - Propofol does not have analgesic properties – always ensure that analgesic agent is also given to the patient for painful procedures.
  - If site injection pain is an issue, may pre-inject site with lidocaine.
  - Hepatic failure – may require lower dosage to be used, as patients may recover more slowly due to decreased elimination.
  - Monitor closely, as level of sedation can easily progress to deep sedation.

Etomidate

- Etomidate is an ultra-short-acting non-barbiturate, non-opioid, non-benzodiazepine sedative-hypnotic.
- It has a rapid onset of action, and short recovery time (comparable to propofol).
- Furthermore, it does not promote histamine release and has minimal effects on the cardiovascular and respiratory systems, making it an appealing option for procedural sedation.
- Dosing:
  - 0.1–0.2 mg/kg IV bolus.
  - 0.05 mg/kg IV for subsequent doses (if necessary).
- Availability and administration:
  - 2 mg/mL – 10 mL ampoule containing 20 mg.
  - Use undiluted.
  - Direct injection IV slowly over 30–60 seconds.
- Onset:
  - <1 minute.
- Duration of action:
  - 3–5 minutes (full recovery 5–15 min).
- Contraindications:
  - Hypersensitivity to etomidate.
- Adverse effects:
  - Transient pain at site of injection (30–80% of patients).
  - Transient myoclonus, uncontrolled eye movements (20–60% of patients).
  - Transient reduction in adrenal cortisol production for 4–8 hours.
  - Transient decrease in cerebral blood flow.
- Monitoring:
  - See Chapter 6 on monitoring during procedural sedation.
  - Signs of adrenal insufficiency (hypotension, hyperkalemia).

- Special considerations:
  - Etomidate is highly irritating, and pre-administration with lidocaine can be considered.
  - Fentanyl decreases etomidate elimination.
  - Premedication with fentanyl or midazolam can reduce myoclonus.

Ketamine

- Ketamine is a phencyclidine derivative that works as an NMDA receptor antagonist and also has been found to bind to opioid mu receptors at higher doses.
- It produces a dissociative state and is a rapid-acting anesthetic with profound analgesic properties.
- It has minimal cardiovascular and respiratory depression.
- Ketamine is able to preserve protective airway reflexes, which may be advantageous when fasting is not assured.
- Unlike other agents that follow the typical sedation continuum, ketamine's dissociative state occurs when a certain dosage threshold is met (usually 1–1.5 mg/kg).
- Safety and efficacy for procedural sedation has been well documented for children.
- A much higher incidence of emergence reactions in the adult population has limited its widespread use.
- Dosing:
  - 1–2 mg/kg IV.
- Availability and administration:
  - 10 mg/mL – 20 mL vial containing 200 mg.
  - 50 mg/mL – 10 mL vial containing 500 mg.
  - Dilute dose to 10 mL with NS.
  - Direct injection IV slowly over 2–3 minutes.
- Onset:
  - 1 minute.
- Duration of action:
  - 5–10 minutes (note analgesic effect outlasts anesthesia effect).
- Contraindications:
  - Hypersensitivity to ketamine.
  - Children <3 months of age.
  - Active pulmonary infection.
  - Cardiovascular disease (angina, heart failure, aneurysm, uncontrolled hypertension).
  - Glaucoma and acute globe injury.
  - History of airway instability, tracheal surgery/stenosis.
  - Psychosis.
  - Porphyria.
  - Thyroid problems.
  - Conditions in which an elevation in BP would be detrimental.

- Adverse effects:
  - Hypertension and tachycardia (more common with rapid administration).
  - May cause hypotension in patients in shock that is catecholamine depleted.
  - Emergence reactions (~12% of adults).
  - Excessive salivation.
  - Transient laryngospasm (0.4%).
  - Nausea and vomiting (~6–7%).
  - Respiratory depression.
- Monitoring:
  - See Chapter 6 on monitoring during procedural sedation.
  - Cardiac function in patients with increased BP or decompensated cardiac function.
- Special consideration:
  - Best suited for short procedures that do not require skeletal muscle relaxation.
  - Pretreatment with a benzodiazepine can potentially reduce emergence reactions by 50%.
  - Benzodiazepines may also blunt sympathomimetic effects of ketamine.
  - Excessive salivation may be treated with atropine or glycopyrrolate (or pretreated to prevent this).
  - Patients experiencing transient laryngospasm may need to be manually bagged (See Chapter 4 on complications of procedural sedation).
  - Avoid in patients who are predisposed to psychotic behavior.
  - Concomitant use of CYP3A4 inhibitors (e.g., azole antifungals, erythromycin, clarithromycin, verapamil, propofol) may increase levels of ketamine.
  - Concomitant use of CYP2C9 inhibitors (e.g., NSAIDs) may increase levels of ketamine.

Fentanyl
- Fentanyl is a highly potent (100 times more potent than morphine) synthetic opioid.
- Opioids are able to provide reliable analgesia.
- Fentanyl has favorable characteristics for use in procedural sedation such as rapid onset, short duration of action, and less cardiovascular depressive effects than the other opioids.
- It also has no active metabolites, and causes much less histamine release (compared to morphine).
- Dosing:
  - 1–1.5 mcg/kg IV initial.
  - Subsequent doses of 1 mcg/kg q 3 minutes.
- Availability and administration:
  - 50 mcg/mL – 2 mL ampoule containing 100 mcg.
  - 50 mcg/mL – 5 mL ampoule containing 250 mcg.

- Use undiluted.
- Direct Inject IV slowly over 15 seconds (avoid "bolus").
- Onset:
  - 1–2 minutes.
- Duration of action:
  - 30–60 minutes.
- Contraindications:
  - Hypersensitivity to fentanyl.
  - Severe respiratory depression or acute respiratory distress (e.g., acute asthma).
  - Increased intracranial pressure.
- Adverse effects:
  - Respiratory depression/apnea.
  - Hypotension.
  - Bradycardia.
  - Muscle and glottic rigidity.
  - Nausea and vomiting.
  - Euphoria.
  - Pruritus.
- Monitoring:
  - See Chapter 6 on monitoring during procedural sedation.
- Special considerations:
  - Inject slowly over at least 15 seconds – Rapid IV injection may cause muscle rigidity, respiratory depression, or cardiovascular collapse.
  - Respiratory depression or excessive sedation can be rapidly reversed with the competitive antagonist naloxone.
  - Symptomatic hypotension may not be fully reversed with naloxone use, as histamine release contributes to hypotension.
  - Pruritus can be managed with antihistamines (e.g., diphenhydramine).
  - Should not be used alone as fentanyl is a pure analgesic.
  - Treat nausea/vomiting with any of the following:
    - Ondansetron 1–4 mg IV.
    - Dimenhydrinate 25–50 mg IV.

Combination Therapy

- Combining agents may increase the risk for adverse effects associated with each drug individually.
- When administering multiple agents, the agent that poses a greater risk of respiratory depression should be administered first.
- The longer acting of the two agents should be administered first.
- A sufficient amount of time should be allowed to pass after administration of the first agent to evaluate its effect prior to administering the second agent.

Fentanyl and Midazolam

- Opioids and benzodiazepines were the first combinations used together for PSA.
- They combine the sedative, amnestic, and anxiolytic properties of benzodiazepines with sufficient analgesic properties of opioids.
- Fentanyl and midazolam have been used in combination effectively for procedural sedation in the emergency department (ED) for many years.
- When combining an opioid and benzodiazepine, the risk of respiratory and cardiac depression increases.
  - Respiratory depression has been observed in up to 25% of patients.
- Titration of dosing to clinical effect can help minimize adverse events.
- Fentanyl should be administered first among the two agents as it poses a greater risk of respiratory depression. The midazolam dose can then be titrated.
- Example of titration:
  - Inject fentanyl 1 mcg/kg IV slowly over 15 seconds.
  - Wait 1 minute.
  - Inject midazolam 0.02 mg/kg IV slowly over 2 minutes.
  - Monitor sedation level.
  - Give additional midazolam 0.02 mg/kg q 3 minutes if needed.

Ketamine and Propofol ("Ketofol")

- The theoretical benefits of this combination include:
  - A rapid onset of sedation and analgesia with a fast recovery time.
  - The sympathomimetic properties of Ketamine should mitigate Propofol-induced hypotension.
  - Propofol might also counteract the nausea and emergence delirium associated with Ketamine.
- Ketamine provides a profound analgesic effect and causes a dissociative state.
- Studies looking at low-dose ketamine used in conjunction with propofol with other agents used in PSA have been difficult to assess due to their small sample size and heterogeneity in regimen and procedures.
- A prospective study demonstrated safely using a low-dose 1:1 ketofol mixture with a median single dose of 0.75 mg/kg ketamine + 0.75 mg/kg propofol (mixed in 1 syringe).
- Adverse events included transient hypoxia, emergence delirium, and insufficient sedation requiring adjunctive doses or medications.

Premedication Agents

Atropine

- Indications:
  - Symptomatic sinus bradycardia.
  - Inhibit salivation or secretions (often caused by ketamine).

- Dose:
  - Bradycardia: 0.5–1 mg q 5 minutes (maximum 2 mg).
  - Treatment or pretreatment for salivation/secretions: 0.4–0.6 mg.
- Availability and administration:
  - 0.4 mg/mL – 1 mL ampoule.
  - 0.6 mg/mL – 1 mL ampoule.
  - 0.1 mg/mL – 10 mL pre-filled syringe containing 1 mg.
  - Use undiluted.
  - Direct Inject IV rapid injection.
- Onset:
  - IV – rapid.
- Contraindications:
  - Hypersensitivity to atropine.
  - Closed (narrow) angle glaucoma.
  - Tachycardia.
  - Obstructive GI disease or ileus.
  - Myasthenia gravis.

Glycopyrrolate
- Indications:
  - Inhibit salivation or secretions (often caused by ketamine).
  - Decrease gastric acid secretion.
- Dose:
  - Treatment or pretreatment for salivation/secretions: 0.04 mg/kg (to a maximum of 0.1 mg).
  - Can be repeated every 3 minutes as needed.
- Availability and administration:
  - 0.2 mg/mL concentration.
- Onset:
  - IV – 1 minute.
- Contraindications:
  - Hypersensitivity to glycopyrrolate.

Reversal Agents
- Reversal agents should not be employed to speed up recovery time, and their routine use should be avoided.
- The duration of action of these agents are often much shorter than the agents that caused the sedation.
  - This can result in an unexpected return of sedation in a seemingly recovered patient.
- Use of reversal agents can also provoke abrupt return of pain or anxiety.

■ Reversal agents should be reserved for prevention of serious complications of procedural sedation agents, such as respiratory depression or cardiorespiratory complications.

Naloxone

■ Naloxone is generally reserved for use to reverse narcotic-induced respiratory depression, apnea, chest wall rigidity, pruritus, and hypotension.
■ Dose:
  ● 0.2 mg IV.
  ● May repeat q 3 minutes.
■ Onset:
  ● IV – 1 minute.
■ Duration of action:
  ● 15–30 minutes.
■ Contraindications:
  ● Hypersensitivity to naloxone.
■ Adverse effects:
  ● Narcotic withdrawal.
  ● Analgesic cessation.

Flumazenil

■ Flumazenil should be reserved for use to reverse serious respiratory depression (in conjunction with assessment of airway and ventilation support if necessary).
■ Benzodiazepine reversal via flumazenil may precipitate seizures in some patients.
■ Flumazenil may also provoke panic attacks in those with underlying panic disorder.
■ Dose:
  ● 0.2 mg IV slowly over 15 seconds.
  ● May repeat at 1-minute interval.
  ● Maximum cumulative dose: 1 mg.
■ Onset:
  ● <1 minute.
■ Duration of action:
  ● 30–45 minutes.
■ Contraindications:
  ● Hypersensitivity to flumazenil.
  ● Use of benzodiazepines to control seizures or increased ICP.
  ● Use with caution in patients who may be dependent on benzodiazepines or alcohol.
■ Adverse effects:
  ● Seizures.
  ● Nausea/vomiting.
  ● Hyperventilation.
  ● Emotional liability, anxiety.
  ● Sweating.

Suggested Reading

American College of Emergency Physicians. Clinical policy for procedural sedation and analgesia in the emergency department. Ann Emerg Med 1998;31:663–677.

American Society of Anesthesiologist Task Force on Sedation and Analgesia by Non-Anesthesiologists. Practice guidelines for sedation and analgesia by non-anesthesiologists. Anesthes 2002;96:1004–1017.

Bond K, Fassbender K, Karkhaneh M, et al. Short-acting agents for procedural sedation and analgesia in Canadian emergency departments: a review of clinical outcomes and economic evaluation [Technology report number 109]. Ottawa: Canadian Agency for Drugs and Technologies in Health, 2008.

Brown TB, Lovato LM, Parker D. Procedural sedation in the acute care setting. Am Fam Physician 2005;71:85–90.

Brunton LL, ed. Goodman and Gilman's the pharmacological basis of therapeutics, 11th ed. New York: McGraw-Hill, 2006.

Falk J, Zed PJ. Etomidate for procedural sedation in the emergency department. Ann Pharmacother 2004;38:1272–1277.

Lacy CF, Armstrong LL, Goldman MP, Lance LL, eds., Drug information handbook, 16th ed. Hudson, OH: Lexi-Comp, 2007.

Lowe G, Dalen D. Low-dose ketamine in addition to propofol for procedural sedation and analgesia in the emergency department. Ann Pharmacother 2007;41:485–492.

Symington L, Thakore S. A review of the use of propofol for procedural sedation in the emergency department. Emerg Med J 2006;23:89–93.

Weaver CS, Hauter WE, Brizendine EJ, et al. Emergency department procedural sedation with propofol: is it safe? J Emerg Med 2007;33:355–361.

Willman E, Andolfatto G. A prospective evaluation of "ketofol" (ketamine/propofol combination) for procedural sedation and analgesia in the emergency department. Ann Emerg Med 2007;49:31–36.

4 Procedural Sedation and Recovery

Alexandra Stefan and Rahim Valani

Introduction

- Ensure that adequate time, personnel, equipment, and location are available for procedural sedation.
- Explain procedure to the patient, and obtain informed consent.
- Consider other options if the PSA procedure is deemed to be unsafe at present:
  - Delay procedure.
  - Scale back targeted depth and use regional anesthesia.
  - Consult anesthesia to have the procedure done in the operating room.
- See Figure 4.1 for overview.

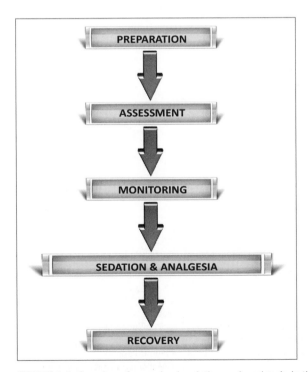

FIGURE 4.1: Overview of procedural sedation and analgesia in the emergency department.

Presedation Assessment

- Informed consent for the procedure:
    - Discuss with the patient all interventions that will be provided, including risks, benefits, potential side effects, and treatment alternatives.
    - Obtaining consent for PSA separate from consent for procedure.
- Document that the risks and benefits of sedation have been discussed.
- Patient assessment:
    - No evidence for routine preprocedural investigations.
    - Complete a thorough history, including anesthesia history and physical exam (see Table 4.1).
- History should include at a minimum:
    - Prior history of cardiac or respiratory illness.
    - Previous adverse events/experience with sedation or general anesthesia (GA).
    - Allergies.
    - Medications.
    - Alcohol/smoking/illicit drug use.
    - Last oral intake.
- Include and document: cardiopulmonary and airway assessment; mental status and baseline vital signs.
- Complete airway assessment is essential to determine suitability for PSA in the emergency department (ED) and potential complications (see Chapter 2).

TABLE 4.1: Patient assessment

History:
- Cardiac/respiratory illness?
- Previous history of general anesthetic?
- Medications/allergies?
- Alcohol/smoking/drugs?
- Last oral intake?

Predictors of difficult airway?
- Previous difficult airway
- Snoring
- Sleep apnea
- Stridor
- Rheumatoid arthritis

Physical exam:
- Vital signs
- Cardiac/respiratory exam
- Body mass index

Predictors of difficult airway:

Head and neck	Jaw	Mouth
Short neck	Macro/retrognathia	Small opening
Limited extension	Trismus	Loose teeth
Hyoid mental distance	Malocclusion	Edentulous
Deformity		Mallampati Grade (see Figure 2.2)

TABLE 4.2: American Society of Anesthesiologists (ASA) physical status classification

Class		Sedation risk
I	Normal, healthy	Minimal
II	Mild systemic disease without functional limitation	Low
III	Severe systemic disease with functional limitation	Intermediate
IV	Severe systemic disease, which is a constant threat to life	High
V	Moribund patient who may not survive without the procedure	Extremely high

- Determine safety of procedural sedation with history and physical examination.
- Patients with ASA physical status class III or greater (see Table 4.2), or those with potential difficult airway should not be done in the ED due to increased risk.

Preprocedural Fasting

- Risk of aspiration with PSA is less likely than in GA.
- Overall risk of 1:3,500 for aspiration and 1:125,000 for subsequent mortality.
- Prospective observational study identified no difference in adverse events between patients classified by preprocedural fasting status.
- No study to date has determined a necessary fasting period before initiation of PSA.
- Guidelines and consensus statements recommend varying fasting periods based on specific substances, that is, solids versus fluids versus clear fluids, but no sufficient evidence to determine absolute recommendations.
- Table 4.3 provides a summary of the guidelines of the American Society of Anesthesiologists, which are a safe and conservative approach.
- Clear liquids ingested up to 2 hours do not adversely affect gastric pH and volume, therefore pose minimal risk.
  - Examples of clear fluids include: water, fruit juice, soda, tea, and coffee.
  - By contrast, particulate matter causes pulmonary damage on aspiration and is thus considered higher risk.

TABLE 4.3: Summary of the American Society of Anesthesiologists preprocedure fasting guidelines

Ingested material	Minimum fasting period (hr)
Clear liquids	2
Breast milk	4
Infant formula	6
Full fluids	6
Light meal	6

Note: These recommendations have been developed for healthy patients undergoing elective surgical procedures.

- Routine administration of antacids does not decrease risk of complications.
- Sedation depth affects likelihood of maintenance of airway reflexes and is thus linked to aspiration risk.
- There is no specific evidence that sedation length in ED affects risk of aspiration.
- Consider timing and depth of PSA in absence of a fasting period.
  - May want to consider delaying the procedure if inadequate fasting period.
- Four-step assessment in the ED:
  - Assess patient risk of aspiration: *standard versus higher risk.*
    - Higher risk includes:
      - Potential for difficult or prolonged ventilation.
      - Extremes of age (>70 years or <6 months).
      - Higher ASA classification.
      - Conditions predisposing to GERD (bowel obstruction, hernia).
  - Assess timing and nature of last oral intake.
  - Assess the urgency of procedure.
- **Emergent:** cardioversion of life-threatening dysrhythmia, reduction of markedly angulated fracture/dislocation, vascular compromise, intractable pain.
- **Urgent:** care of dirty wounds, human bites, hip dislocations, lumbar puncture.
- **Semiurgent:** care of clean wounds, shoulder reduction, foreign body removal.
- **Nonurgent/elective:** ingrown toenail.
  - Determine depth and length of PSA (see Chapter 1 on sedation continuum).

Personnel Requirements Needed for PSA in the ED

- Recognize that the feared complications of PSA include hemodynamic and airway emergencies and thus adequate support must be present.
- PSA at both moderate and deep levels shown to be safe/effective when performed by ED physicians.
- Individual performing moderate/deep sedation must be trained to perform the following:
  - Administer pharmacological agents to desired level of sedation.
  - Monitor patients to maintain desired level of sedation.
  - Manage complications observed during this process.
- No literature evidence on specific number of people that must be present.
  - Current recommendations are to have a support person dedicated to patient monitoring during moderate/deep sedation.
  - Having a separate person doing the procedure.

Equipment and Supplies Necessary for PSA

- Consider the possible complications of PSA when selecting necessary equipment.
  - Allergic reactions.
  - Respiratory arrest.
  - Cardiac arrest.

- Supportive equipment includes:
  - Oxygen.
  - Suction.
  - IV access needed for the procedure and maintained until recovery (this may not be necessary if PSA provided by other routes, such as IM in children).
  - If no IV used, equipment and a qualified person able to establish IV access should be available throughout the procedure.
  - Medications including reversal agents (see Chapter 3).
  - Advanced life-support medications and equipments (including BVM and intubation equipment). See Chapter 2, Airway Assessment and Management for Procedural Sedation, for detailed description.

Monitoring (See Chapter 7)

- Vital signs should be documented including pre- and postprocedure status.
- Monitoring should be targeted to detect early signs of hypotension, bradycardia, apnea, airway obstruction, or hypoventilation.
- Monitor and document (see Chapter 5):
  - Level of awareness as a guide to depth of sedation.
  - Vital signs.

Airway Equipment

- See Chapter 2.

Procedural Sedation

- A variety of pharmacological agents can be used to obtain desired level of sedation (see Chapter 3, Pharmacology of Procedural Sedation).
- The choice of agent depends on:
  - Type of procedure.
  - Desired depth of sedation.
  - Patient factors.
  - Physician comfort with particular agent.
- Slow titration of drugs to the desired effect is essential to minimize complications.
  - Rapid administration is more likely to produce hypotension and respiratory depression.
- Route of administration:
  - Intravenous (IV) administration of sedative analgesic agents increases the likelihood of satisfactory.
  - IV access should be maintained until patient is no longer at risk of complications.
  - If not using IV route for initiation of sedation, consider obtaining IV access after initial sedation.

- Consider and adjust for longer time required for absorption if IM/PO medications before increasing dose by those routes.

Recovery Postsedation: Criteria for Safe Discharge

- Need to monitor adverse events including hypoxemia, apnea, airway obstruction, cardiovascular events, and emesis.
  - These events are generally related to moderate–deep sedation (rate <5%).
- Decreased stimulation, delayed drug absorption, and slow elimination place patients at risk during the recovery period.
- The recovery area should have access to resuscitation equipment.
- It is the responsibility of the physician administering the sedation to ensure that these patients are safe for discharge.
- Duration and frequency of monitoring is individualized; it will depend on:
  - Level of sedation.
  - Overall patient condition.
  - The nature of the intervention.
- Patients should be monitored until they return to baseline mental status and are no longer at risk for cardiorespiratory depression; follow oxygenation, ventilation, and vital sign.
- Guidelines for discharge:
  - The patient is alert and oriented (presedation baseline level).
  - Stable vital signs.
  - Tolerating fluids.
  - Patient is ambulatory.
  - Airway is patent, with protective reflexes intact.
  - Sufficient time postadministration of IV medications.
  - Discharge patients accompanied by a responsible adult and counsel regarding procedure complications.
  - Instructions given to avoid any activity that requires coordination or judgment.
  - Written instruction on when to return to the ED for any complications.

Summary

- Procedural sedation is safe when performed by skilled personnel.
- Strict adherence to presedation assessment, adequate monitoring, and postsedation discharge criteria can decrease risk of complications.

Suggested Reading

Agrawal D, Manzi SF, Gupta PDR, et al. Preprocedural fasting state and adverse events in children undergoing procedural sedation and analgesia in a pediatric emergency department. Ann Emerg Med 2003;42:636–646.

American Society of Anesthesiologists Task Force on Sedation and Analgesia by Non-Anesthesiologists. Practice guidelines for sedation and analgesia by nonanesthesiologists. Anesthesiology 2002;96:1004–1017.

Bahn EL, Holt KR. Procedural sedation and analgesia: a review and new concepts. Emerg Med Clin North Am 2005;23(2):503–517.

Burton JH, Harrah JD, Germann CA, et al. Does end-tidal CO_2 monitoring detect respiratory events prior to current sedation monitoring practices? Acad Emerg Med 2006:13:500–504.

Deltch K, Chudnofsky CR, Dominici P. The utility of supplemental oxygen during emergency department procedural sedation and analgesia with midazolam and fentanyl: a randomized control trial. Ann Emerg Med 2007;49(1):1–8.

Goodwin SA, et al. Clinical policy: procedural sedation and analgesia in the emergency department. Ann Emerg Med 2005;45:177–196.

Green SM, Krauss SB. Pulmonary aspiration risk during emergency department procedural sedation: an examination of the role of fasting and sedation depth. Acad Emerg Med 2002;9:35–42.

Green SM, Roback MG, Miner JR, et al. Fasting and emergency department procedural sedation and analgesia: a consensus-based clinical practice advisory. Ann Emerg Med 2007;49(4):454–461.

Krauss B, Hess D. Capnography for procedural sedation and analgesia in the emergency department. Ann Emerg Med 2007:50(2)177–181.

Miller MA, Levy P, Patel MM. Procedural sedation and analgesia in the emergency department: what are the risks? Emerg Med Clin North Am 2005;23(2):551–572.

Miner JR, Burton JH. Clinical practice advisory: emergency department procedural sedation with propofol. Ann Emerg Med 2007;50:182–187.

Miner JR, Biros MH, Heegaard W, et al. Bispectral electroencephalographic analysis of patients undergoing procedural sedation in the emergency department. Acad Emerg Med 2003;10:638–643.

Roback MG, Bajaj L, Wather JE, et al. Preprocedural fasting and adverse events in procedural sedation and analgesia in a pediatric emergency department: are they related? Ann Emerg Med 2004;44(5):454–459.

5 | Monitoring During Procedural Sedation

Sharon Ramagnano

Introduction

■ All patients undergoing procedural sedation in the emergency department (ED) should have continuous monitoring until ready for discharge.

  ● Continuous monitoring of vital signs and clinical presentation of patient constitute a minimum requirement for patient safety monitoring.

■ Vital signs should include:

  ● Heart rate

  ● Respiratory rate

  ● Blood pressure

  ● Oxygen saturation

■ Capnography is more sensitive for detecting inadequate ventilation/apnea and should now be a standard practice.

Pre-procedural Preparation

■ Staff should ensure that the following equipment is set up in working condition prior to proceeding with the procedure:

  ● Oxygen

  ● Suction

  ● Resuscitation equipment, that is, airway/intubation tray

  ● Hemodynamic monitoring—includes BP, pulse, cardiac monitor, oximetry, and capnography

  ● Sedative reversal agents on hand

  ● Intravenous (IV) access established and maintained

■ The equipment listed in Table 5.1 should be readily available during sedation, while ensuring adequate monitoring of the patient.

Monitoring During the Procedure

■ Appropriate monitoring during procedural sedation is crucial (see Figure 5.1).

■ Monitoring should be targeted to detect early signs of hypotension, bradycardia, apnea, airway obstruction, or hypoventilation.

TABLE 5.1: Equipment necessary during the procedural sedation

Intubation tray	Nasal airway
Various ETT tube sizes	Laryngeal masks
Laryngoscope	Lidocaine spray
Stylette	Emergency crichotomy kit
Tape	Defibrillator
Syringes	Cardiac monitoring
Masks	Continual blood pressure, pulse and oxygen saturation
Ambu bag	Capnography
Suction	Intravenous maintenance
Oxygen	Intravenous fluids
Oral airway	Blood gas syringes

- Regular review and documentation of vital signs is necessary for safe practice.
  - Consensus guidelines recommend recording every 5 minutes once sedation is established.
  - May decrease frequency once patient is awake and alert to the point of discharge.

Clinical Assessment
- No monitoring device replaces clinical assessment of the sedated patient.
- The level of awareness should be used as a guide to depth of sedation.
  - Check response to verbal or painful stimuli, eyelash response, etc. (see Chapter 1).
- Continuous visual inspection of chest-wall motion and air movement is especially important to confirm adequate ventilation.
- Signs of inadequate ventilation should be sought, including:
  - Inadequate or infrequent respirations.
  - Apnea.
  - Cyanosis.
  - Stridor.
  - Snoring.
  - Other signs of upper airway obstruction.
- Monitoring of *respiratory status* has two components: ventilation and oxygenation.
  - Ventilation status can be monitored by clinical observation and auscultation or by capnography, while oxygenation is followed by pulse oximetry.
  - See Chapter 6 on complications related to inadequate oxygenation versus ventilation.

Supplemental Oxygen

- Supplemental oxygen is almost universally applied during procedural sedation in the ED, despite a lack of clinical evidence to support its use.
- It is thought to decrease the incidence and severity of hypoxemia due to airway complications.
  - It may also delay the detection of respiratory depression by pulse oximetry. Therefore, clinical observation of respiratory activity is key.
  - Supplemental oxygen should also be considered when capnography is present.

Pulse Oximetry

- Pulse oximetry provides rapid, noninvasive and continuous estimation of arterial oxygen saturation (SaO_2).
- Its use is universally recommended during procedural sedation, and studies have shown an excellent correlation between arterial hemoglobin oxygen saturation (SaO_2) and pulse oximetry oxygen saturation (SpO_2).
- Although the mechanism of pulse oximetry is complex, a basic understanding allows the recognition of potential limitations.
  - Transmission oximetry is based on differences in the optical transmission of oxygenated and deoxygenated hemoglobin (Hb).
- Advantages:
  - Easy to use.
  - Straightforward interpretation of waveform (see Figure 5.1).
  - No risk to patient.
  - Inexpensive.

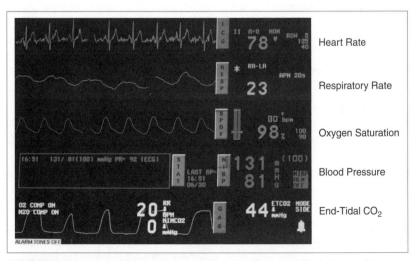

FIGURE 5.1: Standard protocol during procedural sedation should include complete cardiorespiratory and end-tidal CO_2 monitoring.

- Limitations:
  - Falsely *low* SpO$_2$.
    - Hypoperfusion of the extremity.
      - Hypothermia, decreased cardiac output, vasoconstriction secondary to vasopressor use.
    - Movement artifact (e.g., shivering) especially during hypoperfusion.
    - Incorrect sensor application.
    - Highly calloused skin.
    - Artificial nails or nail polish.
    - Presence of abnormal hemoglobin or certain toxins bound to hemoglobin.
      - Methemoglobinemia (reading usually around 85% despite true low or high PaO$_2$).
  - Falsely *elevated* SpO$_2$
    - Carbon monoxide (CO) toxicity.
    - Cyanide poisoning.
      - Reduces oxygen extraction from arterial blood.

Capnography

- Capnography is the measurement of carbon dioxide (CO$_2$) in each breath of the respiratory cycle.
- The capnograph displays a waveform of CO$_2$ measured in mm Hg and the value of CO$_2$ at the end of exhalation, known as the end-tidal CO$_2$ (ETCO$_2$).
- There is a very close correlation, in healthy patients, between ETCO$_2$ and arterial CO$_2$ partial pressure (PaCO$_2$).
  - ETCO$_2$ is ~2–5 mm Hg less than PaCO$_2$.
- Calorimetric monitors use color scales to estimate the range of ETCO$_2$ using pH-sensitive filter paper.

TABLE 5.2: Capnographic changes with common ventilatory patterns during procedural sedation

Ventilatory pattern	Capnographic changes
Periodic breathing	Normal pattern punctuated by apneic pauses May occur with deep sedation
Hypoventilation	High amplitude wide capnogram
Hyperventilation	Low amplitude narrow capnogram
Apnea	Loss of capnogram
Bronchospasm	Curved ascending phase and upsloping of the alveolar plateau

The paper changes from purple (<4 mm Hg CO_2) to tan (4 to 15 mm Hg CO_2) to yellow (>20 mm Hg CO_2).

- This is often used to confirm tube placement following endotracheal intubation.
- Quantitative monitors aspirate samples of gas through a small catheter and are incorporated into nasal prongs or face masks to facilitate CO_2 monitoring during procedural sedation.
  - Limitations include secretion plugging, air leaks, which may dilute the sample, and a 2–3-second delay in response times.
- During procedural sedation, an increase in $ETCO_2$ may be the first sign of inadequate ventilation and has been found to precede a fall in pulse oximetry or clinical signs of respiratory depression.
  - Identifiers of hypoventilation using capnography include:
    - An $ETCO_2$ >50 mm Hg
    - An absent waveform
    - An increase of 10 mm Hg compared to baseline
- It is unclear whether earlier detection of hypercapnia without hypoxemia alters clinical outcome.
- Many conditions affect ventilation perfusion ratios in the lung and can therefore widen the $PaCO_2$–$ETCO_2$ gradient.
  - This results in an inaccurate representation of $PaCO_2$ by $ETCO_2$.
    - Some causes include PE, asthma, cardiac arrest, hypovolemia, and COPD.
    - Although it may not adequately represent $PaCO_2$ in critically ill patients, it is still valuable to detect trends and sudden airway events.
    - For procedural sedation performed in the ED, patients are typically healthy and the $ETCO_2$ should accurately represent the $PaCO_2$.

Recording of Monitored Parameters

- Monitored parameters should be documented at a minimum:
  - Before the beginning of the procedure.
  - After administration of sedative/analgesic agents.
  - On completion of the procedure.
  - During initial recovery.
  - At the time of discharge.
- If recording is performed automatically, device alarms should be set to alert the care team to critical changes in patient status based on the normal preset configuration capabilities.
  - All alarms should be set to *on.*

Staff Availability for Patient Monitoring and Safety

- A designated individual, other than the practitioner performing the procedure, must be present to monitor the patient throughout the procedural sedation and for after care.

- In the ED, a minimum of two staff (nurse, physician, or respiratory therapist) must be available to monitor the patient and assist with the procedure.
- Members of the team must be trained in the recognition of complications associated with IV sedation, specifically:
  - Drug complications/interactions
  - Know the role of pharmacological antagonists
  - Skills in airway management
  - Venipuncture skills
  - Arrhythmia recognition

Post-procedure Monitoring

- Patients should be observed until they are no longer at increased risk for cardiorespiratory depression.
- Vital signs and respiratory function should be monitored at regular intervals until patients are suitable for discharge.
- Discharge according to specified criteria with verbal and written discharge instructions (see Chapter 4).
- Staff must ensure that a complete discharge instruction sheet or information is provided to the patient and family.
- The discharge instructions should include at a minimum:
  - Procedure performed
  - Medications received pre-, during, and post-procedure
  - Any prescriptions required post-discharge
  - Any adverse events that occurred during the procedure
  - After care for the presenting problem that the patient arrived with
  - When to return to the family physician for follow-up and when to return to the ED if required
  - Instructions regarding dressing changes/cast care/suture removal, etc.
  - Tetanus status (if given ensure that this information is provided for the patient to alert their family physician for their medical records)

Suggested Reading

Godwin SA, Caro DA, Wolf SJ, et al. Clinical policy: procedural sedation and analgesia in the emergency department. *Ann Emerg Med* 2005;45:177–196.

Jubran A. Pulse oximetry. In: Tobin MJ, ed. Principles and practice of intensive care monitoring. New York: McGraw-Hill, 1998.

Krauss B, Hess DR. Capnography for procedural sedation and analgesia in the emergency department. *Ann Emerg Med* 2007;50(2):172–181.

6

Adverse Events and Complications of Procedural Sedation

Angela Stone and Mark Freedman

Overview

- The complication rate of procedural sedation is estimated to be <1% in the hospitals and specialties routinely practicing procedural sedation and analgesia.
  - Adverse event rate is estimated at 2%–3% in pediatric patients.
  - The most common complication is respiratory depression and airway obstruction.
  - Medication errors.
- Many of the complications related to PSA can be prevented by:
  - Appropriate monitoring and recognition of respiratory depression or arrest.
  - Adequate monitoring.
  - Ensuring the correct dose of medications (avoid drug calculation error).
  - Careful titration of medications.
  - Appropriate patient assessment.
  - Avoiding drug–drug interactions.
  - Personnel present who are trained in airway management and resuscitation.
  - Management of potential complications requires early recognition. Therefore, clinical observation and appropriate monitoring during the procedure is essential in order to identify and treat possible adverse effects (see Chapter 5).
- Most complications during procedural sedation can be managed noninvasively.

Propofol

Respiratory Depression

- Propofol causes dose-related apnea and respiratory depression.
- No clinically significant events reported in studies with PSA, with most cases managed by bag-valve mask ventilation.
- Recognition of respiratory depression is essential.
  - Managed with jaw thrust, repositioning of the airway, or assisted ventilation for a brief period.
  - The need for intubation after the use of propofol in the emergency department (ED) has not been reported.

- Propofol is reported to have the lowest rate of respiratory depression when compared with methohexital, fentanyl/midazolam, and etomidate.

Hypotension

- Propofol commonly results in a drop in blood pressure, which is often transient.
- More commonly seen with rapid bolus, for example patients who are hypovolemic, or have poor cardiovascular reserve.
- When compared with etomidate, propofol has been found to induce greater hypotension, although this is transient and of unknown clinical significance.
- Can be treated with Trendelenburg positioning, fluid bolus, or short-acting vasopressor (phenylephrine).

Injection Pain

- Injection pain has been reported in up to 70% of patients.
- Warning the patient often alleviates anxiety when pain is felt with the injection.
- Lidocaine, either mixed with propofol (1 mL of 1% lidocaine in 19 mL propofol) or given with a rubber tourniquet in place 30–120 s before injection (0.5 mL/kg) has been found to prevent injection pain.

Ketamine

Laryngospasm

- Rare but potentially life-threatening side complication.
- Unrelated to age, sex, underlying medical condition, or dose.
- Associated with procedures that stimulate hyperactive gag reflex through direct instrumentation or secretions appear to represent a higher risk.
- Risk factors include:
  - Upper airway infection.
  - Age between 3 and 12 months.
  - Active pulmonary disease including asthma.
- Laryngospasm often manifests as hypoxia and decreased chest wall movement not responsive to maneuvers to open the upper airway.
- Consider bag-valve mask and positive pressure ventilation as first line approach – breaks most cases of laryngospasm.
  - In severe circumstances may require urgent paralysis and intubation.

Hypersalivation

- Ketamine stimulates salivary and tracheobronchial secretions.
- In children, coadminister with atropine (0.01 mg/kg; min 0.1 mg, max 0.5 mg) or glycopyrrolate (0.005 mg/kg; max 0.25 mg).
- The use of atropine appears to be unnecessary in adult patients in the ED.

Nausea and Vomiting

- Vomiting occurs in 0%–9% of patients receiving ketamine.
- In children, the incidence appears to be age-related, with a higher risk in patients aged 5 years and older.

- Vomiting most often occurs during the late recovery phase when the patient is awake and alert.
- Protective airway reflexes are maintained during dissociative anesthesia with ketamine, therefore, significant aspiration is extremely rare.
  - Ketamine is therefore preferred over other agents for urgent or emergent procedures when fasting is not assured.
- Delayed vomiting may occur after discharge, and patients should be informed about this (see Chapter 4 on discharge instructions).

Clonus and Hypertonicity
- Ketamine does not produce muscle relaxation, and random purposeless movements, hypertonicity, and clonus are not unusual.
- These movements are usually unrelated to painful stimuli and do not need to be treated.

Sympathomimetic Effects
- Ketamine inhibits the reuptake of catecholamines, resulting in mild to moderate increases in blood pressure, heart rate, and myocardial oxygen consumption.
- Potential risk to patients with coronary artery disease.
  - Actual risk is unknown due to limited experiences in this population of patients.

Emergence Phenomenon
- Ketamine is associated with a hallucinatory "emergence reaction" known as emergence delirium.
- It occurs in up to 30% of adult patients and is much less common in children.
- Risk factors:
  - Age >16 years.
  - Female sex.
  - Rapid IV administration.
  - Use of large doses.
- Hallucinations can be pleasurable or more commonly frightening like nightmares.
  - Use of benzodiazepines concurrently with ketamine is believed to blunt, but not entirely eliminate this reaction in adults.
  - In pediatric patients, unpleasant recovery reactions are uncommon and are typically mild. There is no evidence to suggest the use of prophylactic administration of benzodiazepines in this population.
  - Consider their use only when treating unpleasant emergency reactions, should they occur.

Ketamine and Propofol (Ketofol)
- Ketofol is a mixture of both ketamine and propofol used to achieve procedural sedation.

- The reasoning behind using both agents is that they are theoretically synergistic.
  - The sympathomimetic properties of ketamine should mitigate propofol-induced hypotension.
  - Propofol might also counteract the nausea and emergence delerium associated with ketamine.
- The most common dosing mixture is a 1:1 combination of both drugs at doses of 0.50–0.75 mg/kg (10 mg/mL).
  - Propofol and ketamine can be used simultaneously yet from separate syringes thus allowing their independent titration.
- The pitfall of this combination is that ketamine lacks the dose-dependent progressive effect typical of propofol.
- The dose used in most studies (0.75 mg/kg) is considered subdissociative, not achieving its characteristic trancelike state, and acts instead like a simple analgesic.
  - Dissociative doses of ketamine are usually between 1.0 and 1.5 mg/kg IV.
- Studies have shown that the combination is effective and appears safe for procedural sedation.
- Adverse events included transient hypoxia, emergence delirium, and insufficient sedation requiring adjunctive doses or medications.

Etomidate

Respiratory Depression

- A brief period of apnea may occur following etomidate administration.
  - Risk factors include:
    - Rapid administration (<80 sec).
    - Higher doses (>0.2 mg/kg).
    - Older patients (>55 years of age).
- At typical procedural sedation doses, respiratory depression is rare and if it does occur is usually transient and mild.
- No studies have reported the need to intubate a patient after its use in procedural sedation.

Myoclonus

- Myoclonus is a characteristic and common side effect of etomidate occurring anywhere from 0%–21% of cases.
- It usually lasts <1 minute and can be minor and focal or severe and associated with full body rigidity, tonic clonic activity, hypoventilation, and hypoxia.
- Myoclonus-induced respiratory depression has not been reported with ED use.

Nausea and Vomiting

- The incidence of nausea and vomiting with etomidate ranges from 0%–5%.
- The risk of nausea and vomiting appears to be dose-related and is generally not a problem with doses used for procedural sedation.
- There have been no documented cases of aspiration.

- Randomized controlled trial comparing propofol to etomidate found that etomidate induced vomiting more frequently than that seen with propofol use during procedural sedation.

Adrenal Suppression

- Etomidate is known to cause adrenal suppression, even following a single dose.
  - The mechanism is via inhibition of 11-beta-hydroxylase activity.
- Unlikely of any clinical significance in the setting of PSA.

Pain on Injection

- Pain on injection is most likely caused by the propylene glycol solvent.
- Methods to decrease discomfort include:
  - Using larger veins.
  - Mixing 1 cc of 1% lidocaine with each 10 mL of etomidate.
  - Flushing with saline.
  - Pretreating with fentanyl.

Midazolam

Respiratory Depression

- Midazolam causes central respiratory depression through decreased sensitivity to carbon dioxide.
- It is dose-dependent, peaking at 3 minutes after IV administration.
- More pronounced in:
  - Elderly patients.
  - Patients with COPD.
  - When coadministered with other respiratory depressants.
- Consider reduced dosage in patients with COPD and in patients older than 60 years.

Prolonged Sedation

- Most commonly occurs in elderly patients.
- Reversal of the sedating effects of benzodiazepines is achieved using flumazenil, which is benzodiazepine antagonist with an onset of action of 1–2 minutes.
  - It is given as an IV titration starting with a bolus of 0.5 mg in adults followed by 0.1 mg until a desired response is achieved.
  - Can precipitate seizures in patients who are benzodiazepine dependent. Consider noninvasive support of ventilation until patient's respiratory status improves.

Paradoxical Agitation

- Paradoxical reactions to benzodiazepines are occasionally seen in young children.
- Reactions include agitation, combativeness, and inconsolability.
- Treatment is supportive with airway and blood pressure management.

- Flumazenil has been shown to be quick acting and effective in abating paradoxical reactions in children.
  - Starting dose of 0.01 mg/kg (up to 0.2 mg).
  - It may be repeated to achieve the desired level of consciousness to a maximum dose of 1.0 mg or 0.05 mg/kg.
- Haloperidol may be a safe alternative to flumazenil but is less commonly used due to its risk of extrapyramidal side effects.

Fentanyl

Respiratory Depression

- Fentanyl reduces the responsiveness of the brain-stem respiratory center to carbon dioxide.
- Maximal respiratory depression occurs 5 minutes after intravenous administration.
- The magnitude is dose dependent and is intensified by the coadministration of other respiratory depressants, particularly midazolam.

Muscular and Glottic Rigidity

- Occurs only with high doses of fentanyl and has never been reported with its use in the ED for PSA.
- Management includes reversal with naloxone or paralysis with succinylcholine.

Seizures

- Also associated with high doses and has not been reported in ED patients.

Pruritus

- Mild facial pruritus is common.
- There is little or no histamine release with fentanyl use, therefore anything more serious (urticaria or anaphylactoid reactions) are seldom seen.

Midazolam and Fentanyl

- The key to avoiding complications is the titration to a desired effect.
- The combination of drugs may accentuate the potential side effects of each.
- Because opioids pose a greater risk of respiratory depression, it has been suggested that when using in combination with a benzodiazepine the opioid should be given first and the benzodiazepine titrated to effect.

Summary

- Adverse event rates for PSA in the ED are low, and most can be managed noninvasively.
- The most common complication of PSA is respiratory depression.
- Different medications used for PSA have adverse reactions and complications that can be managed.

Suggested Reading

Falk J, Zed PJ. Etomidate for procedural sedation in the emergency department. Ann Pharmacother 2004;38:1272–1277.

Godwin SA, Caro DA, Wolf SJ, et al. Clinical policy: procedural sedation and analgesia in the emergency department. Ann Emerg Med 2005;45(2):177–196.

Green SM. Research advances in procedural sedation and analgesia. Ann Emerg Med 2007;49(1):31–36.

Loh G, et al. Low-dose ketamine in addition to propofol for procedural sedation and analgesia in the emergency department. Ann Pharmacother 2007;41(3): 485–492.

Marx JA, Hockberger RS, Walls RM, et al. Rosen's emergency medicine: concepts and clinical practice, 6th ed. Philadelphia, PA: Mosby, 2006.

Miner JR, Danahy M, Moch A, et al. Randomized clinical trial of etomidate versus propofol for procedural sedation in the emergency department. Ann Emerg Med 2007;49:15–22.

Schenarts CL, Burton JH, Riker RR. Adrenocortical dysfunction following etomidate induction in emergency department patients. Acad Emerg Med 2001;8:1–7.

Willman EV, Andolfatto G. A prospective evaluation of "ketofol" (ketamine/propofol combination) for procedural sedation and analgesia in the emergency department. Ann Emerg Med 2007;49:23–30.

7

Pediatric Procedural Sedation
Savithiri Ratnapalan

Pediatric Procedural Sedation and Analgesia

- Procedural sedation is the technique of administering a single drug or a combination of drugs with sedative, analgesic, or dissociative properties to induce a state that allows children to:
  - Tolerate painful or unpleasant procedures
  - Stay still for some non-painful procedures
- The most common reasons for pediatric procedural sedation are:
  - Orthopedics (most common, and includes fracture reductions, dislocations, and immobilization/splinting)
  - Laceration repair
  - Foreign body removal
  - Lumbar puncture
  - CT scans

Challenges in Children

- Assessing the level of sedation in a child may be harder than in adults.
  - A child can easily move from moderate sedation to general anesthesia with minimal increases in sedative agents.
- Children come in various sizes and need age-appropriate equipment.
  - Ensure age- and size-appropriate equipment, including:
    - ▶ Blood pressure cuffs for different ages.
    - ▶ Doppler blood pressure monitors.
    - ▶ Pulse oximetry probes.
    - ▶ Intravenous canula.
    - ▶ Airway equipment – masks, resuscitation bags, and intubation equipment.
- Children range from neonates to teenagers, and need specific dose calculations.
  - Obtain accurate weight of patient of appropriate dosing.
  - Drug doses should be calculated and checked by at least two healthcare professionals.
  - Most common cause of drug error is dose inaccuracies.

- Children should come with a parent or guardian.
  - Consent from the parent and assent from child (as appropriate) should be obtained before the procedure.
- Children need simple explanations and clear instructions.
- Children need a calm monitored environment for procedural sedation and for recovery.

Pediatric Characteristics That Need Consideration

- Young infants have relatively less oxygen reserve (greater oxygen consumption).
  - Hypoxemia occurs more rapidly.
  - Appropriate size bag and mask ventilation should be available.
- Pediatric patient sizes may vary from 2.5–100 kg. The "pediatric crash cart" is bigger and should have age-appropriate equipment.
- Airway sizes may vary unpredictably among pediatric patients of same age and weight.
- At times, three different-sized endotracheal tubes should be available for the patients of the same age (the calculated size and a size smaller and larger).
  - The appropriate uncuffed endo-tracheal-tube size may be determined by the following formula (age in years):
    - $4 + (1/4)$ (age)
    - Subtract 0.5 for the appropriate size cuffed ETT
      - For example, for a 4-year-old child: uncuffed ETT size = $4 + (1/4)4 = 5$
      - So, cuffed ETT size = $5 - 0.5 = 4.5$.
  - The appropriate depth of ETT insertion can be approximated by:
    - Over 1 year of age:
      - Oral: $13 + (1/2)$age
      - Nasal: $15 + (1/2)$age
    - Infants (weight in kg):
      - Oral: $8 + (1/2)$(weight)
      - Nasal: $9 + (1/2)$(weight)
- Small children have small airways.
  - Since resistance to air flow is inversely proportional to the fourth power of the radius of the airway, 1 mm of concentric edema in a newborn trachea (radius ~2 mm) increases resistance about 16 times.
  - The presence of upper respiratory tract infection should be assessed prior to sedation, adjuvant agents to reduce secretions may have to be used, and vigilance in airway monitoring observed.
- There are anatomic differences between the infant and the adult upper airway:
  - Infant larynx:
    - More superior in neck.
    - Epiglottis shorter, angled more over glottis.
    - Vocal cords slanted: anterior commissure more inferior.
    - Larynx cone-shaped: narrowest at subglottic cricoid ring.
    - Softer, more pliable: may be gently flexed or rotated anteriorly.

- Infant tongue is relatively larger.
- Infant head is relatively larger: naturally flexed in supine position.
- Caution in intubation: extension of head may result in tracheal extubation, while flexion may lead to main stem intubation.

- Young infants (less than approximately 2–3 months) are obligate nose breathers.
- Infants and young children have limited hepatic glycogen storage and are more prone to hypoglycemia when fasted for prolonged periods.
  - Consider starting an intravenous maintenance fluid such as D5% N Saline if the child has fasted or is expected to fast for a long period.
- Gastroesophageal reflux is common in infants. Watch out for vomiting post sedation.

Policies and Protocols for a Safe Pediatric Sedation Within the ED

- Trained personnel in pediatric sedation and airway management.
- Accurate weight measurement, drug dose calculations, and a protocol mandating two persons sign-off on drugs.
- Age-appropriate equipment to monitor and manage potential adverse effects of sedation in children.
- Preprinted orders and monitoring sheets should be a requirement for any department performing PSA.
- Documentation of consent.

Exclusion Criteria and Contraindications for ED Pediatric Sedation

Patient Criteria

- ASA classification >II.
- History of known airway problems: snoring, obstructive sleep apnea, large tonsils or adenoids, tracheomalacia, tracheostenosis, congenital abnormalities involving the airway (e.g., Down syndrome, Pierre Robin syndrome, Treacher Collins syndrome, and Crouzon's disease).
- Cardiovascular disease: repaired or unrepaired congenital heart disease and congestive heart failure.
- Severe neurologic disease, severe hypotonia, and evidence of increased intracranial pressure.
- Severe renal or liver disease.
- Severe gastroesophageal reflux and previous esophageal surgery or injury.
- Patients at increased risk of pulmonary aspiration of gastric contents (e.g., full stomach).
- Potential neck injury, limitations in moving neck/opening mouth/jaw movement.
- History of known sedation failure.
- Home oxygen therapy/or home ventilation.
- Sickle cell disease.
- Baseline vital signs indicate SaO_2 <95% in room air.

Procedure Criteria

■ Sedation time greater than 30 minutes

Provider/Facilities Criteria

■ Lack of personnel experienced in pediatric sedation and airway management
■ Lack of resuscitation drugs or age-appropriate equipment
■ Lack of monitoring facilities during recovery
■ Lack of an experienced physician to do the procedure and/or supervise the procedure

Commonly Used Drugs and Combinations

■ Various single and combination drugs have been used with good safety profiles.
■ See Table 7.1.

Choice of Drugs

■ Sedative drugs used and the depth of sedation needed depend on the patient characteristics and procedures.
  ● Patient characteristics: age, fasting status, comorbid conditions, maturity, level of cooperation and level of anxiety.
  ● Procedures: painless or painful, severity of pain, urgency of the procedure, level of complexity, how much motion control is needed, and length of the procedure.

Adverse Reactions and Complication

■ See Chapter 6.
■ Type 1 IgE-mediated allergic reaction to procedural sedation is unusual.

TABLE 7.1: Sample medications that can be used for procedural sedation in pediatric patients

Level of sedation	Drug choices
Mild	Midazolam PO, Intranasal
	Nitrous oxide
Moderate	Midazolam IV
	Etomidate IV
	Midazolam IV and Fentanyl IV ± nitrous oxide
Moderate to deep sedation	Propofol
Dissociative sedation	Ketamine

- More common reactions are:
  - ▶ Histamine release (Morphine, Meperidine).
  - ▶ Nasal pruritus (Fentanyl).
  - ▶ Paradoxical reactions (Benzodiazepines, Barbiturates).
  - ▶ Emergence reactions to Ketamine.
  - ▶ Laryngospasm reported with both Ketamine and Propofol.
- Children experience higher rates of respiratory depression and hypoxia than adults.
- Adverse events in children occur more frequently in:
  - Younger children.
  - Sedation performed in non-hospital-based facilities.
  - With the use of three or more drugs or drugs with long half-lives.

Commonly Used Pharmacologic Agents for Procedural Sedation and Analgesia in Children

Midazolam

- Short-acting benzodiazepine.
- Provides sedation, anxiolysis, and amnesia (*no* analgesic effects).
- Minimal hemodynamic effects (mild hypotension with compensatory tachycardia).
- Dose- and infusion-dependent respiratory depression and apnea especially with opioids (Table 7.2).

Nitrous Oxide

- Provides anxiolysis, amnesia, and mild analgesia.
- Noninvasive, rapid onset, short duration of action.
- Generally used in concentrations of 20%–50% mixed with oxygen.
- Free flow nitrous oxide versus demand valve (Entonox®)– 50% nitrous/ 50% oxygen.
- Scavenging device essential.
- Indications: minor procedures, for example, intravenous access, laceration repair, burn debridement, and as an adjunct for more painful procedures, for example, fracture reduction.

TABLE 7.2: Midazolam dosing in pediatric patients

Route of administration	Dose
Oral	Weight <20 kg, 0.5–0.75 mg/kg
	Weight >20 kg, 0.3–0.5 mg/kg (max 20 mg)
Intranasal	–0.1–0.3 mg/kg (max 1 mL)
Intravenous	0.05–0.15 mg/kg titrate slowly to effect

■ Avoid in patients with pneumothorax, bowel obstruction, intracranial injury, and cardiovascular compromise.

Ketamine

■ Dissociative agent that produces a trance-like cataleptic state.
  ● Profound analgesia.
  ● Amnesia.
  ● Retention of protective airway reflexes, spontaneous respirations, and cardiopulmonary stability.
■ *Indications:* Procedures requiring profound analgesia and immobility, for example, fracture reduction and complex laceration repair.
■ Most commonly used agent for procedural sedation in children.
■ Significant side-effect profiles including:
  ● Increased intracranial pressure.
  ● Hypersalivation.
  ● Tachycardia.
  ● Hypertension.
  ● Nystagmus and diplopia.
  ● Muscle hypertonicity.
  ● Emesis.
  ● Transient apnea or respiratory depression.
  ● Laryngospasm.
■ Relative contraindications:
  ● Head injury associated with altered mental status.
  ● Loss of consciousness or emesis.
  ● Cardiovascular disease.
  ● Glaucoma or acute globe injury.
  ● Psychosis.
  ● Thyroid disorder.
  ● Age <3 months.
  ● Procedures involving stimulation of posterior pharynx and active pulmonary infection or disease (URI).
■ Dosing for ketamine is given in Table 7.3.

TABLE 7.3: Dosing of ketamine for procedural sedation in pediatric patients[a]

	Intravenous	Intramuscular
Dosage	1–1.5 mg/kg	4 mg/kg
Onset of action	1–2 min	5–10 min
Duration of action	10–15 min	15–30 min

[a]May be used in conjunction with adjuvant agents including atropine or glycopyrrolate and/or midazolam.

Drug-Specific Considerations in Pediatrics

- Any sedative but specifically chloral hydrate:
  - Prolonged sedation and airway obstruction.
- Midazolam:
  - Paradoxical reactions in 20% of children with oral midazolam.
  - Intravenous midazolam can be titrated and this reaction is not common.
- Ketamine:
  - Hypersalivation. Young children may need adjuvant drugs such as Atropine or Glycopyrrolate.
- Propofol:
  - Hypotension may not be associated with tachycardia and could be missed if not measured.

Pearls to Avoid Adverse Events in Pediatric Patients

- Choose your patient:
  - Take a good history.
  - Identify those with upper respiratory infections, significant underlying physical illnesses, obstructive airway disease, psychosis, and drug allergy.
  - Avoid sedating any child with severe systemic disease (ASA ≥3).
- Know the drugs you use:
  - Accurate weight of the child.
  - Dosage should not only be weight-dependent, but also age- and disease-dependent.
  - Know your upper limits for each drug and its potential side effects.
  - Draw your own drugs and label them.
- Monitor patients carefully:
  - Continuous cardiac monitoring and pulse oximetry plus independent observer who checks vital signs.
  - Continue monitoring until patient returns to baseline.
  - Be cautious of increased sedation after painful stimulus is removed and vomiting during recovery.
- Fully prepare for any complications before starting the procedure.
  - Age-appropriate resuscitative equipment, reversal agents, and skilled personnel in advanced pediatric life support should be immediately available.

Steps for Procedural Sedation and Analgesia

- Refer to Chapter 4.

Summary

- Customize the sedation technique for the patient and the procedure to be performed.

- Ensure appropriate personnel and interactive monitoring.

- Potential for adverse outcomes may increase when three or more sedating medications are used. Knowledge of each drug's time of onset, peak response, and duration of action is essential.

- Drugs with longer duration of action require longer periods of observation. This concept is important for infants and toddlers transported in car safety seats.

Suggested Reading

American Academy of Pediatrics. Guidelines for monitoring and management of pediatric patients during and after sedation for diagnostic and therapeutic procedures: An update. Pediatrics 2006;118:2587–2606.

American Academy of Pediatrics, Committee on Drugs. Guidelines for monitoring and management of pediatric patients during and after sedation for diagnostic and therapeutic procedures: Addendum. Pediatrics 2002;110:4:836–38.

American Society of Anesthesiologists. Practice guidelines for sedation and analgesia by non-anesthesiologists. Anesthesiology 2002;96:1004–1017.

Cravero JP, Bilke GT. Review of pediatric sedation. Anesth Analg 2004;99(5): 1355–1364.

Cravero JP, Blike GT, Beach M, et al. Pediatric sedation research consortium incidence and nature of adverse events during pediatric sedation/anesthesia for procedures outside the operating room. Report from the Pediatric Sedation Research Consortium. Pediatrics 2006;118(3):1087–1096.

Godwin SA, Caro DA, Wolf SJ, et al. Clinical policy: procedural sedation and analgesia in the emergency department. Ann Emerg Med 2005;45(2):177–196.

Hoffman GM, Nowakowski R, Troshynski TJ, et al. Risk reduction in pediatric procedural sedation by application of an American Academy of Pediatrics/ American Society of Anesthesiologists process model. Pediatrics 2002;109: 2:236–243.

Krauss B, Green SM. Sedation and analgesia for procedures in children. N Engl J Med 2000;342:(13);938–945.

Mace SE, Barata IA, Cravero, JP, et al. Clinical policy: evidence-based approach to pharmacological agents used in pediatric sedation and analgesia in the emergency department. Ann Emerg Med. 2004;44:342–377.

Mace SE, Brown LA, Francis L, et al. Clinical policy: critical issues in the sedation of pediatric patients in the emergency department. Ann Emerg Med 2008;51(4):378–399.

Zempsky WT. Cravero JP, Committee on Pediatric Emergency Medicine and Section on Anesthesiology and Pain Medicine. Relief of pain and anxiety in pediatric patients in emergency medical systems. Pediatrics 2004;114:5:1348–1356.

Pain Management and Regional Anesthesia

8

Introduction to Pain Management

Jeff Gadsden

Epidemiology of Pain Presentation

- Pain is the most common presenting complaint to the emergency department (ED).
  - In France, pain-related issues account for 67% of the presenting complaints.
- Pain is initially assessed 90% of the time but reassessments occur less frequently (48% on discharge).
  - For those assessed on discharge, 27% still had pain (8% severe).
- Delay for pain management is related to ED volumes, lack of triage nurses (especially in small departments), and initial pain intensity.
- Pain intensity follow-up is important to assess to determine analgesic effectiveness.
- Patient satisfaction is related to earlier effective pain management.
- Quality indicators for pain management include
  - Time to first dose of analgesic in all painful conditions.
  - Percentage of patients with documented pain assessment.
- The mean **expectation** for time to analgesic administration for ED patients is 23 minutes, compared with actual mean time to analgesic administration of 78 minutes.

Concepts in Pain Management

- Multimodal pain management is better than any one agent alone.
  - Adding acetaminophen to ibuprofen, for example, is better than either agent alone.
  - As well, both can be given to complement narcotic therapy.
- Dosing intervals should be according to the earliest allowable time to avoid loss of pain control and optimize pharmacokinetics (see Chapter 10).
- Once nausea is controlled, oral options for analgesics should be explored to facilitate early conversion.
- For people presenting with acute on chronic pain, management should take into consideration their current daily opiate consumption.
- "Muscle relaxants," such as Robaxacet (acetaminophen/methocarbamol) and Flexeril (cyclobenzaprine), have little evidence to support their use.

- Neuropathic pain is a challenging issue.
- May need to consider the use of nontraditional analgesics, for example, pregabalin, amitriptyline, or gabapentin.
- Consider regional nerve blocks.
  - Intercostal nerve blocks have been shown to be beneficial in rib fractures.
  - See Chapter 12.
- Prior studies have suggested that protocol-driven analgesia can be more effective than provider initiated analgesia.
- Protocolized analgesic administration facilitates a greater percentage of patients being treated in a timely fashion and should be part of every ED with appropriate supporting infrastructure.

Anatomy and Physiology of Pain

Acute Pain

- Acute pain is defined as "pain of recent onset and probable limited duration. It usually has an identifiable temporal and causal relationship to injury or disease."
- Also, it can be thought of as "physiological pain" or "useful pain."
- In contrast, chronic pain typically lasts beyond time of healing and frequently has no identifiable cause.
- Acute and chronic pain in fact may represent a continuum rather than two separate entities.

Peripheral Receptors and Afferent Fibers

- Axons of primary afferent nerves end in skin, subcutaneous tissue, periosteum, joints, muscles, and viscera.
- There are *no* specialized pain receptors: free nerve endings (nociceptors) are sensitive to noxious physical stimuli.
  - These respond to chemical, mechanical, or thermal energy that threatens the integrity of the tissue.
- There are two main types of nociceptive afferents:
  - Aδ-fiber mechanothermal nociceptors:
    - ▶ Thinly myelinated (therefore, faster than unmyelinated C-fibers)
    - ▶ Responds to heat, cold, and pressure
    - ▶ Provides "first pain" information critical for protective withdrawal reflex
  - C-fiber polymodal nociceptors:
    - ▶ Unmyelinated (slow)
    - ▶ Respond to a broad range of physical (heat, cold, pressure) and chemical stimuli
    - ▶ Provides "second pain" that is classically burning in nature
- Tissue damage (e.g., trauma, infection, inflammation, or ischemia) disrupts cell structure and promotes the release of an "inflammatory soup" of chemical mediators that activate and/or sensitize nearby C-fibers (e.g., protons, bradykinin, histamine, prostaglandins, serotonin, and substance P).

■ Most tissues have both types of nociceptors; exceptions include liver, brain, and lung tissue which have no afferent pain fibers.

Visceral Referred Pain

■ Occasionally, axons from visceral afferent nerve converge onto the same second-order neuron as somatic afferents.

■ The brain is unable to distinguish between the two inputs and projects the sensation to the somatic structure.

   ● Examples: myocardial ischemia felt as aching pain in left shoulder; gallbladder distention felt as pain in right shoulder.

Pain Transmission

■ Mechanical or chemical signals are converted first to action potentials in the periphery.

■ Conducted along first-order neurons to the dorsal horn of the spinal cord.

■ Synapse with second-order neurons and ascend to thalamus via the spinothalamic and spinoreticular tracts.

■ Project to a number of areas including

   ● Periaqueductal gray matter, an area rich in opioid receptors

   ● The somatosensory cortex

   ● The frontal lobes

   ● The hypothalamus

■ This variety of destinations is congruent with the idea of pain as a complicated process that involves sensory, emotional, and social aspects.

Central Sensitization (Windup)

■ Following trauma in the periphery, the dorsal horn exhibits enhanced responsiveness to further stimuli, a phenomenon termed "windup."

■ Caused by continued barrage of nociceptive input to dorsal horn neurons and a gradual increase in spinal cord neuronal activity.

■ This results in an increased responsiveness to normally innocuous mechanical stimuli (allodynia) and a zone of hyperalgesia in uninjured tissue surrounding the site of injury.

■ Loco-regional techniques (e.g., nerve blocks) that interrupt the barrage of afferent input effectively prevent windup if provided early and for the appropriate duration (see Chapter 12).

■ Windup can also be partially modulated by the use of NMDA-receptor antagonists (i.e., ketamine).

Modulation of Pain

■ The experience of pain can be modulated by cortical events such as high levels of stress, distraction, or intense excitement (e.g., in battlefield or sporting injuries).

■ The release of endogenous opioids (endorphins) is thought to be responsible for these occurrences.

- Similarly, anxiety or depression can enhance the experience of pain for a given stimulus and may be related to reduced discharge of descending inhibitory pathways.
- The gate theory of pain modulation (Melzack and Wall) states that the transmission of impulses into the dorsal horn is controlled by a spinal gating system.
- This is controlled by the relative activity in large or small fibers.
- Activity in large fibers tends to inhibit transmission, whereas small fiber activity stimulates transmission (i.e., opens the gate).
- The coincident flooding of the dorsal horn with cutaneous touch and pressure sensation may close the gate for smaller nociceptive input (Figure 8.1).

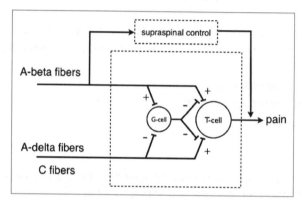

FIGURE 8.1: The gate control theory of pain. The gate cell (G-cell) is capable of modulating the activity of the afferent activity to the transmitter cell (T-cell). Input from large, nonnociceptive fibers (e.g., A-beta fibers carrying touch and pressure impulses) activates the gate, which prevents further input from nociceptive afferents. There are also cortical and subcortical inputs that influence the gate mechanism.

Progression of Acute to Chronic Pain

- The continuum of acute to chronic pain:
  - Chronic pain is increasingly being referred to as "persistent pain."
  - Patients with chronic pain often relate onset of their pain to an acute injury.
  - Chronic pain is common after surgical procedures (see Table 8.1).
  - Increasing recognition that nervous system exhibits remarkable plasticity – consistent afferent nociceptive input can result in permanent neurophysiologic change.
- Preventive analgesia.
  - Defined as the persistence of analgesic treatment efficacy beyond its expected duration.
  - Refers to the minimizing of central sensitization and windup by the provision of quality analgesia that is continued for as long as the sensitizing stimulus persists.

TABLE 8.1: Incidence of chronic pain after surgery

Type of operation	Incidence of chronic pain (%)
Amputation	30–85
Thoracotomy	5–65
Mastectomy	11–57
Inguinal hernia	5–63
Cesarean section	6–55
Coronary artery bypass	30–50

- Most effectively achieved by the use of multimodal analgesia.
- The following have all been shown in meta-analyses to be effective in minimizing the incidence of persistent pain:
  ▶ Gabapentin
  ▶ Local anesthetics (i.e., nerve blocks, epidural analgesia)
  ▶ Nonsteroidal anti-inflammatory drugs
  ▶ NMDA antagonists (e.g., ketamine, dextromethorphan)
- The combination of multiple agents allows for complementary modes of action while reducing the dosage (and therefore side effects) of any one individual agent.

Adverse Physiological Effects of Acute Pain

Acute Pain and the Injury Response
- Acute pain activates the neurohumoral and immune response to injury.
- This is an adaptive survival response that, if prolonged, can have adverse effects on outcome.
- The hormonal/metabolic response includes increased cortisol, catecholamines and glucagon, and decrease in insulin sensitivity.
- As pain is one of the major triggers of the injury response, and the duration of the response is related to the duration of the stimulus, effective pain relief can have a significant impact on these adverse consequences.

Adverse Physiologic Effects (See Figure 8.2)
- Hyperglycemia is proportional to the extent of the injury response.
- Injury leads to upregulation of membrane glucose transport proteins glut-1, 2, and 3 which are located in brain, endothelium, liver, and some blood cells.
- Results in cellular glucose overload, glycosylation of proteins such as immunoglobulins, and production of oxygen free radicals.
- Lipolysis results in increased free fatty acids which depress myocardial contractility and increase myocardial oxygen consumption.

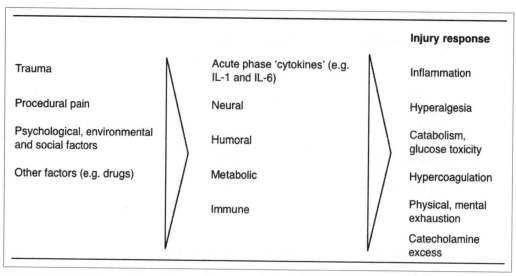

FIGURE 8.2: The injury response.

- Accelerated protein breakdown and amino acid oxidation lead to a negative nitrogen balance and poor wound healing, impaired immune function, and diminished muscle strength.
- Pain activates sympathetic efferent nerves causing increases in heart rate, inotropy, and blood pressure and increasing risk for myocardial ischemia.

Pharmacogenomics and Acute Pain

- Susceptibility to pain conditions appears to have genetic variability.
- Correlation of gene expression with a drug's efficacy of toxicity can lead to optimization of analgesic therapy.

Loss of Pain Sensation

- Hereditary syndromes exist in association with loss of pain sensation.
- Example: "channelopathy-associated insensitivity to pain," caused by a variant in the voltage-gated sodium channel. These individuals cannot propagate action potentials on peripheral nerves and are unable to feel pain.
- Other familial peripheral and autonomic neuropathies have been described such as hereditary sensory and autonomic neuropathy type IV (HSAN-4), a severe autosomal recessive disease characterized by childhood onset of insensitivity to pain and anhidrosis.

Reduced Sensitivity to Pain

- Associated with variants in genes encoding the mu-opioid receptor, catechol-O-methyl-transferase (COMT), and transient receptor potential ($TRPV_1$).
- These patients frequently report increased pain scores and require greater than usual doses of opioid analgesics.

Drug Metabolism

- Drug metabolizing enzymes are a major target for identifying associations between an individual's genetic profile and drug response.
- The CYP2D6 gene is highly polymorphic and influences the metabolism of codeine, oxycodone, and tramadol.
  - For example, CYP2D6 genotypes predicting ultra-rapid metabolism resulted in about 50% higher plasma concentrations of morphine and its glucuronides following oral codeine compared with the normal population.
  - Morphine toxicity and death have been reported in a breastfed neonate whose mother was an ultra-rapid metabolizer of codeine.
  - Similarly, 1%–3% of Caucasians are poor metabolizers of NSAIDs such as ibuprofen and naproxen; these patients are at risk for increased adverse effects from elevated blood levels of the parent drug.

Summary

- Pain is a common presentation to the ED.
- Adequate assessment and management of pain is an important part of patient care.

The author would like to thank Mark Mensour and Andrew Healey for their contributions to this chapter.

Suggested Reading

Bisgaard T, Klarskov B, Rosenberg J, et al. Characteristics and prediction of early pain after laparoscopic cholecystectomy. Pain 2001;90(3):261–269.

Carlson JD, Maire JJ, Martenson ME, et al. Sensitization of pain-modulating neurons in the rostral ventromedial medulla after peripheral nerve injury. J Neurosci 2007;27(48):13222–13231.

Chapman CR, Tuckett RP, Song CW. Pain and stress in a systems perspective: reciprocal neural, endocrine, and immune interactions. J Pain 2008;9(2): 122–145.

Cousins MJ, Power I, Smith G. 1996 Labat lecture: pain – a persistent problem. Reg Anesth Pain Med 2000;25(1):6–21.

Evans E, Turley N, Robinson N, et al. Randomised controlled trial of patient controlled analgesia compared with nurse delivered analgesia in an emergency department. Emerg Med J 2005;22:25–29.

Fosnocht D, Swanson E, Barton E. Changing attitudes about pain and pain control in emergency medicine. Emerg Med Clin North Am 2005;23(2):297–306.

Hunt SP, Mantyh PW. The molecular dynamics of pain control. Nat Rev Neurosci 2001;2(2):83–91.

Kehlet H, Jensen TS, Woolf CJ. Persistent postsurgical pain: risk factors and prevention. Lancet 2006;367(9522):1618–1625.

Møiniche S, Kehlet H, Dahl JB. A qualitative and quantitative systematic review of preemptive analgesia for postoperative pain relief: the role of timing of analgesia. Anesthesiology 2002;96(3):725–741.

Sandkühler J. Models and mechanisms of hyperalgesia and allodynia. Physiol Rev 2009;89(2):707–758.

Stein C, Clark JD, Oh U, et al. Peripheral mechanisms of pain and analgesia. Brain Res Rev 2009;60(1):90–113.

Williams DG, Patel A, Howard RF. Pharmacogenetics of codeine metabolism in an urban population of children and its implications for analgesic reliability. Br J Anaesth 2002;89(6):839–845.

9   Chronic Pain Management in the ED

Rahim Valani

Introduction

- Chronic pain is defined by the International Association for the Study of Pain as pain without the biological value that has persisted beyond the normal healing time.
  - Usually defined as pain lasting for more than 6 months.
- It is estimated that 35% of the US population suffer from chronic pain, which costs $40 billion per year.
- Approximately 21% of people with chronic pain are dissatisfied with their current pain management.
- Stages of progression from acute to chronic pain:
  - Stage 1 – acute phase.
    - Initial psychological distress that is expected – fear and anxiety.
  - Stage 2 – exacerbation of psychological problems.
    - When pain lasts over 2–4 months.
    - Patient's response includes anger, distress, and somatization.
    - Social, financial, and environment factors play an important role in how the patient copes with this phase.
  - Stage 3 – acceptance of the "sick role."
    - Physical deconditioning occurs in all three stages.
- The most common chronic pain conditions in general practice include:
  - Irritable bowel syndrome.
  - Osteoarthritis.
  - Lower back pain.
  - Chronic pelvic pain.
  - Migraine headaches/tension headaches.
  - Fibromyalgia.
- It is important to complete a thorough pain history for every patient who presents to the ED, including:
  - Pain characteristics – onset, location, quality, radiation, severity, temporal profile, and alleviating factors.

- Effects on daily living – Can they cope with daily activities of living such as bathing, dressing themselves, doing the laundry, and cooking?
- Effects on their family/friends.
- Effects on their employment – Are they able to continue to work? What are the limitations? Can they be accommodated for limited duties?
- Changes in recreational activities.
- Psychological impact of pain – mood, sexual function, sleep, etc.

- Physical examinations should include:
  - Inspecting for:
    - Signs of inflammation.
    - Trophic changes.
    - Deformities.
  - Range of motion of affected joints and muscles.
  - Palpation for tenderness, crepitus, and warmth.

- Issues surrounding the adequate treatment of chronic pain:
  - Poor knowledge by health care professionals.
  - Inadequate pain assessment.
  - Not recognizing multidimensional cause of pain.
  - Poor documentation.
  - Misconceptions about the use of opioids.
  - Patient's reluctance to report pain.

- Opioid used for non-cancer and chronic pain.
  - Opioids continue to be one of the most prescribed medications for chronic pain.
  - Three largest increases over the 10 years (1997–2006) include the use of:
    - Methadone (1,177% increase).
    - Oxycodone (732%).
    - Fentanyl (479%).

- Consider the following steps in prescribing opioids for chronic pain:
  - Comprehensive initial evaluation.
  - Establish need for opioid, either as a supplemental medication or lack of response to prior medication.
  - Assess risk of starting and using opioid medication.
  - Establish treatment goals with patient.
  - Obtain informed consent and agreement with patient.
  - Initial dose adjustment phase in first 3 months, followed by frequent reevaluation to titrate dose accordingly.
  - Outcomes – dose adjustments, steady state, or discontinuing medications.

- Consequences of chronic pain:
  - Inability to perform normal activities of daily living.
  - Feeling of hopelessness.
  - Fear of activities that can exacerbate the pain.

Myofascial Pain

- Estimated to affect up to 54% of individuals.
- Regional painful muscle/soft tissue condition related to specific trigger points and related pain.
  - Also referred to as myofascial trigger point pain.
- Hallmark is localized trigger points with focal tenderness.
  - Usually tight bands typically located in the center of the rigid muscle.
  - Pain on sustained compression over the tender point.
  - Local twitch response within the band of muscle on plucking palpation across the fibers.
- Immediate response to injection of local anesthetic is characteristic.
- Classified as primary or secondary.
  - Primary – from a specific cause with ongoing pain with continued use of that muscle.
  - Secondary – pain referred from a primary site due to mechanical stress or inflammation.
- Common posterior myofascial trigger points are located at:
  - Levator scapulae.
  - Trapezius.
  - Rhomboids.
  - Quadratus lumborum.
  - Piriformis.
- Etiology:
  - Posttraumatic.
  - Chronic repetitive injuries.
  - Muscle wasting – malignancy and stroke.
  - Muscle ischemia – arterial obstruction.
  - Environmental – heat- or cold-related injuries.
- Differential diagnosis includes:
  - Non-myofascial trigger point (fibromyalgia):
    - Myofascial trigger point patients have fewer systemic complaints compared to patients with fibromyalgia.
  - Musculoskeletal diseases – tendinitis, arthritis, and occupational myalgia.
  - Systemic diseases – arthritides (rheumatic, psoriatic), infection.
  - Psychiatric.
  - Drug reaction.
- Chronic myofascial pain can persist after the acute event due to:
  - Dorsal horn neural plasticity.
  - Ongoing self-perpetuating ischemic changes.
  - Development of circuits from the trigger point to the spinal cord.
  - Prognosis is directly related to the duration of symptoms.

- Treatment options:
  - Any pharmacotherapy must be done in conjunction with physical therapy for best results.
  - Primary treatment is to restore functional activity through performance and stretching exercises.
    - Spray with cool vaporizer followed by muscle stretches.
    - Deep pressure soft tissue massage.
    - Post-isometric relaxation. (The muscle is in a stretched position with isometric contraction against minimal resistance. This is followed by relaxation and a gentle stretch.)
    - Reciprocal inhibition.
  - Non-steroidal anti-inflammatory drugs (NSAIDs).
  - Injection of local anesthetic to trigger point site.
  - Other adjuncts: ultrasound, iontophoresis, TENS, and thermotherapy.
  - Botulinum toxin A injection.

Fibromyalgia

- Chronic pain condition that involves muscles and myofascial tissues, accompanied by trigger points.
- Prevalence is estimated at 1%–3% in the general population and is more common in females aged between 20 and 50 years.
- Pathophysiology is poorly understood.
- American College of Rheumatology definition:
  - Generalized pain involving three or more sites for 3 months or longer.
  - Exclude other conditions.
  - Reproducible pain over 11 of the 18 fibromyalgia tender points.
- Treatment should incorporate:
  - Patient education.
  - Other medications to control non-pain symptoms such as depression.
  - Aggressive use of cognitive-behavioral approaches.
  - Pharmacological treatments include:
    - Analgesics – NSAIDs and opioids.
    - Antidepressants:
      - 5HT and norepinephrine are the main neurotransmitters involved.
      - TCAs and SNRIs (Venlafaxine, Duloxetine, Milnacipran) seem to be most effective in treating fibromyalgia.
    - Alpha2-delta ligands:
      - Gabapentin and Pregabalin limit neuronal excitation and enhance inhibition.
    - Growth hormone:
      - Evidence that about one-third of patients with fibromyalgia have a functional growth hormone deficiency.

- Nonpharmacological treatments:
  - ▶ Physical therapy.
  - ▶ Movement and exercises.
  - ▶ Cognitive behavioral treatments.
  - ▶ Complementary/alternative treatment.

Complex Regional Pain Syndrome

- Incidence varies from 5.5–26.2 per 100,000.
- It is more common in women and with increasing age (peaks in the fifth to seventh decade).
- Categorized as type I (no nerve lesion identified) and type II.
  - Type I is more common.
  - Type I was formerly known as "reflex sympathetic dystrophy."
- Pain out of proportion to the inciting event is characteristic.
- Fractures are the most common precipitating event, and usually in the upper limb.
  - Increased pressure and complaints of cast tightness during cast immobilization are predictors of complex regional pain syndrome (CRPS).
- Symptoms are varied:
  - Inflammation.
  - Impaired motor function.
  - Trophic changes.
- Exact etiology is complex, and includes:
  - Autonomic (sympathetic) nervous system hyperactivity:
    - ▶ Increased sweating.
    - ▶ Trophic changes.
    - ▶ Extreme vasoconstriction.
    - ▶ Coldness in the limb.
  - Somatic nervous system:
    - ▶ Pain and sensory disturbances.
  - Inflammation.
  - Hypoxia:
    - ▶ Decreased capillary oxygenation.
    - ▶ Elevated lactate levels.
    - ▶ Extreme vasoconstriction.
  - Psychological factors.
- Treatment options:
  - Glucocorticoids.
  - NSAIDs – usually primary therapy.
  - GABA agonists – Baclofen is an option for dystonia associated with CRPS.
  - Bisphosphonates – benefit on pain, swelling, and mobility.

Whiplash-Associated Disorder

- Caused by an acceleration–deceleration mechanism of energy transfer of the neck.
- Incidence is estimated at 70–328 per 100,000 in Canada and the USA.
- Most patients improve within the first 3 months.
- It is the most common cause of neck pain associated with musculo-ligamentous conditions.
- The Quebec Task Force grades of whiplash-associated disorder (WAD):
  - Grade 0 – no neck symptoms or physical signs.
  - Grade 1 – neck pain, stiffness, or tenderness; no physical signs.
  - Grade 2 – neck symptoms and musculoskeletal signs (decreased range of motion and point tenderness).
  - Grade 3 – neck symptoms and neurological signs (decreased or absent deep tendon reflexes, muscle weakness, sensory deficits).
  - Grade 4 – neck symptoms with fracture or dislocation.
- Chronic pain develops in 15% to 20% of whiplash injuries.
- Chronic pain and disability are complex presentations due to injury-related factors (physical) and psychosocial factors (event-related factors).
- The Quebec Task Force defined late whiplash syndrome as presence of pain, restriction of motion, or other symptoms at 6 months or more after the injury.
  - Hinders activities of daily living.
    - Subcategories include:
      - Local cervical syndrome.
      - Cervicogenic headaches.
      - Cervicogenic vertigo.
      - Cervico-brachial syndrome.
      - Behavioral manifestations.
- Predictors of poor prognosis include:
  - High baseline neck pain intensity.
  - Presence of headache.
  - High WAD Grade.
  - Lack of secondary education.
- Characteristics of collision (rear-ended, side impact, frontal), gender, and age are not clear indicators of poor prognosis.
- Assessment and management based on WAD-Plus Model:
  - Grade of WAD.
  - Time since injury.
  - Pain experience.
  - Chronicity factors – depends on socioeconomic status, prior medical status, symptom severity, psychosocial factors, use of health care, and compensatory factors.
- Abnormal central pain processing has implications for management of myofascial trigger points and tight bands.

- Manual therapy and exercise are effective noninvasive interventions for neck pain.
- Interventional treatments include:
- Steroid injection in epidural space, trigger points, or facet joints:
  - Botulinum toxin injection to muscle trigger points.
  - Percutaneous radiofrequency treatment.
  - Chiropractic care can improve cervical range of motion and pain in the management of WAD.

Suggested Reading

Abram S, Haddox JD. The pain clinic manual. Philadelphia, PA: Lippincott Williams & Wilkins, 2004.

Banks C, Mackrodt K. Chronic pain management. London: Whurr Publishers, 2005.

Bennett R. Myofascial pain syndromes and their evaluation. Best Pract Res Clin Rheumatol 2007;21(3):427–445.

Bruehl S. An update on the pathophysiology of complex regional pain syndrome. Anesthesiology 2010;113:713–725.

Cummings M, Baldry P. Regional myofascial pain: diagnosis and management. Best Pract Res Clin Rheumatol 2007;21(2):367–387.

De Mos M, Sturkenboom CJM, Huygen F. Current understanding of complex regional pain syndrome. Pain Pract 2009;9(2):86–99.

Gatchel RJ. Clinical essentials of pain management. Washington, DC: American Psychological Association, 2005.

Gupta A, Mehdi A, Duwell M, et al. Evidence-based review of the pharmacoeconomics related to the management of chronic non-malignant pain. J Pain Palliat Care Pharmacother 2010;24:152–156.

Hubbard JE. Myofascial trigger points: what physicians should know about these neurological imitators. Minn Med 2010;93(5):42–45.

Latrigue AM. Myofascial pain syndrome: treatments. J Pain Palliat Care Pharmacother. 2009;23(2):169–170.

Lavelle ED, Lavelle W, Smith HS. Myofascial trigger points. Anesthesiol Clin 2007;25: 841–851.

Manchikanti L, Datta S, Vallejo R, et al. Opioids for noncancer pain. Expert Rev Neurother 2010;10(5):775–789.

Sarzi-Puttini P, Atzeni F, Cazzola M. Neuroendocrine therapy of fibromyalgia syndrome: an update. Ann N Y Acad Sci 2010;1193;91–97.

Warfield CA, Bajwa Z. Principles and practice of pain medicine. Toronto: McGraw-Hill, 2004.

Pharmacology of Pain Management

Leanne Drehmer

Pharmacology of Pain Management

- Numerous classes of medications are available for the treatment of pain, and the treatment can be tailored depending on the nature and severity of pain (i.e., acute pain, chronic pain, and neuropathic pain).
- An effective choice of medication for treating pain should include consideration of:
  - Allergies or sensitivities to medications.
  - Recent or previous history of pain medication used (what worked, what has not worked, and why).
  - Formulations of medications available (i.e., oral liquids, oral tablets, sustained-release oral tablets, injectables, and topicals).
  - Appropriate dosing, dose conversions, and relative potency.
- Ineffective management of acute pain can not only lead to patient/caregiver dissatisfaction, but also may potentially lead to progression to chronic pain.
- Classes of medications used for the management of pain include:
  - Non-opioid analgesics.
  - Opioid analgesics.
  - Co-analgesics/adjunctive agents.
  - Topical anesthetics.

Non-opioid Medications

- Non-opioid medications are used for the treatment of mild to moderate pain.
- The most common non-opioids are acetaminophen and nonsteroidal anti-inflammatory drugs (NSAIDs).

Acetaminophen

- Acetaminophen is a non-opioid analgesic that also has antipyretic properties, used for mild to moderate pain, and for fever.
- Acetaminophen inhibits synthesis of prostaglandins in the central nervous system (CNS), and inhibits peripheral pain signal neurotransmission.
- As an antipyretic, acetaminophen acts on the heat-regulating center in the hypothalamus, inducing vasodilation and sweating to disperse body heat.

- Routes: oral (PO) or rectal (PR).
- Dosing:
  - PO: 10–15 mg/kg/dose q4h PRN.
  - PR: 10–20 mg/kg/dose q4h PRN.
- Onset: PO – 15 minutes, PR – 30 minutes.
- Peak effect: PO – 30–60 minutes, PR – 2 hours.
- Duration: PO/PR – 4–6 hours.
- Pharmacokinetics:
  - Well absorbed orally, slower absorption and effect rectally.
  - Metabolized in liver via glucuronidation, and by P450 enzyme CYP2E1 to metabolite NAPQI (hepatotoxic in acute overdose).
  - Excreted by the kidneys.
- Contraindications:
  - Liver dysfunction, hypersensitivity to acetaminophen.
- Significant drug interactions:
  - Phenytoin, barbiturates (i.e., phenobarbital), and carbamazepine may decrease the levels and effect of acetaminophen.
  - Minor increase in bleeding risk with warfarin.
- Adverse effects:
  - Nausea/vomiting (may take with food).
  - Rash.
  - Hepatotoxicity with chronic use or acute overdose.
  - Renal injury with chronic use.
- Monitoring:
  - Pain and/or fever reduction, liver enzymes and liver function tests (LFTs) with chronic use.
- Acetaminophen special considerations and pearls:
  - Lack of action on prostaglandins in the peripheral nervous system (PNS) likely related to lack of anti-inflammatory action.
  - No gastric irritation/ulceration compared to NSAIDs.
  - Extended-release 650-mg tablets also available, but usually not used for acute pain in children.
  - Caution different concentrations of oral drops (80 mg/mL) versus oral liquid suspension (32 mg/mL).
  - Be aware that acetaminophen is a component of multiple over-the-counter and prescription products, limit acetaminophen content from all sources to ≤75 mg/kg/day.
  - Ensure that the foil is removed from suppositories prior to insertion; half doses should be achieved by cutting suppositories lengthwise symmetrically.
  - PR absorption is slower and less complete than oral absorption (see dosing above).
  - Oral liquid may be instilled rectally (limit volume to 80 mg/1 mL).

Nonsteroidal Anti-inflammatory Drugs

- NSAIDs are used for treatment of mild to moderate pain.
- NSAIDs inhibit the peripheral synthesis of inflammatory prostaglandins, and have analgesic, anti-inflammatory, and anti-pyretic properties.
- Typical NSAIDs used in the pediatric population are ibuprofen, naproxen, and ketorolac.
- Routes: PO, PR; IM/IV (ketorolac).
- Dosing:
  - Ibuprofen: PO – 5–10 mg/kg/dose PO q6–8h.
  - Naproxen: PO – 5–10 mg/kg/dose PR BID PRN.
    - ▶ Rectal dosing: less than 50 kg–250 mg/dose PR, greater than 50 kg–500 mg/dose PR (maximum 1,000 mg/day).
  - Ketorolac: IV/IM/PO 0.5 mg/kg/dose q6h PRN (see special considerations below; maximum 15–30 mg/dose).
- Administer PO with food to decrease stomach irritation.
- Onset: PO – 30–60 minutes, PR – 2 hours, IM/IV – 30 minutes.
- Peak effect: PO – 2–4 hours, PR – 4 hours, IM/IV – 2–3 hours.
- Duration – PO/PR/IM/IV – 6–8 hours.
- Pharmacokinetics:
  - Well absorbed orally, slower absorption rectally.
  - Metabolized by liver, eliminated by kidneys.
- Contraindications:
  - Hypersensitivity to NSAIDs.
  - Severe asthma triggered by NSAID use.
  - Acute active bleeding.
  - Elevated bleeding risk.
- Significant drug interactions:
  - Anti-platelet agents, anticoagulants, steroids (ASA, clopidogrel, warfarin, prednisone, etc. – additive bleeding risk).
  - Anti-hypertensive medications (ACE inhibitors, B-blockers – reduced anti-hypertensive effect).
  - ACE inhibitors, diuretics (increased risk of hyperkalemia).
  - NSAIDs may increase the levels of aminoglycosides (i.e., gentamicin), cyclosporine, digoxin, haloperidol, lithium, methotrexate, quinolones (i.e., ciprofloxacin), and vancomycin.
  - Levels and effects of NSAIDs may be increased by tricyclic antidepressants (i.e., amitriptyline), selective serotonin reuptake inhibitors (SSRIs) (i.e., fluoxetine), serotonin/norepinephrine reuptake inhibitors (SNRIs) (i.e., venlafaxine), and probenecid.
- Adverse effects:
  - GI irritation/nausea/vomiting/heartburn (take with food).
  - Rash and pruritus.
  - Dizziness.
  - Fluid retention.

- Monitoring:
  - Reduction of pain/fever/inflammation.
  - Blood pressure/edema for cardiac patients.
  - Liver enzymes/LFTs, CBC, and renal function for chronic use.
- NSAID special considerations and pearls:
  - Relative increasing potency of NSAIDs generally ibuprofen → naproxen → ketorolac.
  - Naproxen helpful in rheumatic or inflammatory disorders.
  - Ketorolac to be used parenterally IV or IM if patient not able to tolerate other PO NSAIDs, and to be used short term only (i.e., <5 days) due to GI irritation/bleeding risk. The IM route is also painful.
  - May transition to PO ketorolac if needed, but preferred to use ibuprofen as PO agent.

Opioid Medications

Codeine

- Codeine is an opioid analgesic inhibiting neurotransmission in the ascending pain pathway, and an antitussive (in lower doses), acting centrally on the medulla.
- Codeine is a *pro-drug*, which does not have significant pharmacological activity until metabolized by cytochrome P450 CYP2D6 enzymes in the liver to the active metabolite, morphine (~10% metabolized to active morphine).
- Codeine should be used with caution for pediatric pain management due to variable pharmacokinetics and unpredictable efficacy and toxicity.
- Routes of administration: PO, IM, subcutaneous (Subcut).
- Dosing:
  - PO analgesia: 0.5–1 mg/kg/dose q4–6h PRN.
  - PO antitussive: 0.15–0.3 mg/kg/dose q4–6h PRN.
  - IM/Subcut: 0.5–1 mg/kg/dose q4–6h PRN.
  - Maximum analgesic dose: 1.5 mg/kg/dose, or 60 mg/dose.
  - Maximum antitussive dose: 20 mg/dose.
  - Adjust dose for renal impairment.
  - Sustained-release products used for chronic pain and dosed based on average daily requirements of immediate-release preparations, usually dosed q12h.
- Product availability and administration:
  - PO liquid: codeine phosphate – 5 mg/mL.
  - PO *immediate-release* tablets: codeine phosphate – 15 and 30 mg.
  - PO *sustained-release* tablets (for chronic pain): codeine contin (codeine sulfate trihydrate) – 50, 100, 150, and 200 mg.
  - IM/Subcut: 30 mg/mL ampoule q4–6h PRN.
  - IM or Subcut no dilution required, do not administer IV.

- Onset: PO – 30–60 minutes; IM/Subcut – 10–30 minutes.
- Peak effect: PO – 60–90 minutes (4 hours for sustained release); IM/Subcut – 30–60 minutes.
- Duration: PO and IM/Subcut – 4–6 hours (12 hr for sustained-release PO tablets).
- Pharmacokinetics:
  - Readily absorbed orally, ~60% bioavailability (see Section IV: PO Conversion, Table 10.3).
  - Low protein binding.
  - Metabolized by CYP2D6 in liver into morphine-active metabolite.
  - Eliminated primarily by the kidneys.
- Contraindications:
  - Hypersensitivity/allergy to codeine or morphine.
- Significant drug interactions:
  - Other CNS depressant/respiratory depressant medications (i.e., other opioids and benzodiazepines).
  - Quinidine (inhibits CYP2D6, decreased effect of codeine).
- Adverse effects:
  - Excessive sedation.
  - Respiratory depression.
  - Bradycardia.
  - Hypotension.
  - Dizziness.
  - Drowsiness.
  - Constipation.
  - Urinary retention.
  - GI upset (may take with food).
- Monitoring:
  - HR, RR, BP, reduction in pain score, level of sedation and constipation.
- Codeine special considerations and pearls:
  - Respiratory depression can occur even at therapeutic doses (not necessarily only at toxic doses).
  - Codeine does not necessarily have less adverse effects than stronger opioids.
  - Genetic polymorphism – variable pharmacokinetics and unpredictability.
    - P450 CYP2D6 enzyme that metabolizes codeine to morphine for therapeutic effect is highly polymorphic.
    - Up to 28% of North African, Ethiopian, or Saudi Arabian patients; 10% of Caucasian patients; 3% of African American patients, and 1% of Chinese, Japanese, or Hispanic patients are "ultra-metabolizers" – meaning more than expected codeine is metabolized to morphine (excessive sedation, respiratory depression, or even death may result).
    - "Slow or poor metabolizers," on the other hand, may experience ineffective pain relief with codeine.

- Genetic testing for CYP2D6 polymorphism is not readily commercially available, thus it is preferential to prescribe oral or parenteral morphine directly (rather than producing morphine indirectly through codeine metabolism).
- IV administration of codeine is not recommended due to significant histamine release and potential for severe vasodilation, hypotension, and cardiac/respiratory arrest.
- IM/Subcut administration of codeine is also not recommended as painful and poorly tolerated.
- Multiple combination products containing codeine are available; be aware of potential for additive sources of codeine.
- Prescribed in mg, not mL for oral liquids.
- Do not crush sustained-release products used for chronic pain.
- Consider stool softener or mild laxative to mitigate constipation.

Morphine

- Morphine binds to the μ-opioid receptors in the CNS, inhibiting neurotransmission in the ascending pain pathway.
- Routes of administration: PO, IV, IM/Subcut, and PR.
- Dosing:
  - Intermittent parenteral doses: 0.05–0.1 mg/kg/dose IV/IM/Subcut q2h PRN.
  - Intermittent oral/rectal doses: 0.2–0.5 mg/kg/dose PO/PR q4h PRN.
  - Continuous infusion: 0.1 mg/kg IV bolus loading dose, then 10–40 mcg/kg/hr IV/Subcut infusion, with 0.1 mg/kg/dose q1h PRN for breakthrough pain.
  - Sustained-release products used for chronic pain and dosed based on average daily requirements of immediate-release preparations.
  - Adjust dose in renal impairment.
- Product availability and administration:
  - PO liquid: morphine – 1 mg/mL.
  - PO immediate-release tablets: 5, 10, 20, 25, 30, 40, 50, and 60 mg.
  - PO q12h sustained-release tablets (MS-Contin): 15, 30, 60, and 100 mg
  - PO q24h sustained-release capsules (Kadian): 10, 20, 50, and 100 mg.
  - PO extended-release capsules (M-Eslon): 15, 30, 60, and 100 mg.
  - Suppository: 5, 10, 20, and 30 mg.
  - Injectable: 2, 10, and 50 mg/mL.
  - Inject slowly over 2 minutes, dilute with NS or D5W to a maximum concentration of 5 mg/mL (rapid IV administration may produce excessive histamine release, hypotension, respiratory/cardiac depression). Ensure respiratory support is readily available.
  - Wean continuous infusions slowly to prevent withdrawal syndrome.
  - For chronic pain, sustained-release capsules may be opened and sprinkled on food (pellets to be swallowed whole).
- Onset: PO/PR – 30 minutes (60 minutes for controlled-release PO preparations); IV/IM/Subcut: 5 minutes.

- Peak effect: PO/PR – 60 minutes (~4 hr for controlled-release PO preparations); IV/IM/Subcut – 10–20 minutes.
- Duration: PO/PR – 4 hours (12 hr for controlled-release PO preparations); IV/IM/Subcut – 3–4 hours.
- Pharmacokinetics:
  - Good oral absorption, bioavailability ~40% (see Section IV: PO conversion section, Table 10.3).
  - Moderate protein binding.
  - Morphine is the active metabolite of codeine (via CYP2D6), and also produces active metabolite (morphine-6-glucuronide) when morphine is metabolized in the liver by glucuronidation (does not involve P450 CYP enzymes).
  - Eliminated primarily by the kidneys.
- Contraindications:
  - Hypersensitivity/allergy to morphine or codeine.
- Significant drug interactions:
  - Other CNS depressant/respiratory depressant medications (i.e., other opioids, benzodiazepines).
  - Morphine may increase levels of SSRIs, thiazide diuretics.
  - Succinylcholine, amphetamines, and antipsychotics may increase the levels/effects of morphine.
  - MAO inhibitors may increase the effect of morphine.
- Adverse effects:
  - Excessive sedation.
  - Respiratory depression.
  - Bradycardia.
  - Hypotension.
  - Dizziness.
  - Drowsiness.
  - Pruritus.
  - Constipation.
  - Urinary retention.
  - GI upset (may take PO with food).
- Monitoring:
  - HR, RR, BP, oxygen saturation, reduction in pain score, level of sedation, and constipation.
- Morphine special considerations and pearls:
  - Preservative-free morphine is available for epidural or intrathecal use.
  - High-alert medication for medication errors associated with abbreviations – not to be prescribed as MSO_4 for morphine sulfate (interchange error with magnesium sulfate – $MgSO_4$).
  - Prescribe in mg, not mL for oral liquid.
  - Do not crush sustained-release products for chronic pain.
  - Consider stool softener or mild laxative to mitigate constipation.

Fentanyl

- Synthetic opioid analgesic (increased potency compared to morphine), which is short acting.
- Binds to μ-opioid receptors in CNS to inhibit ascending pain pathways.
- It has sedative and analgesic properties.
- Routes of administration: IV/IM/Subcut, intranasal, and topical patch.
- Dosing:
  - IV/IM/Subcut intermittent: 0.5–1 mcg/kg/dose q1h PRN.
  - IV continuous infusion: 1–2 mcg/kg bolus, then 0.5–3 mcg/kg/hr, with 1–2 mcg/kg/dose q1h PRN for breakthrough pain.
  - Transdermal patch: change q72h (moderate to severe chronic pain, with stable opioid requirements; not for opioid naïve patients): conversion of stable opioid dose to equivalent dose of fentanyl in consultation with pharmacist – individualize dosing.
  - Intranasal: 1.5 mcg/kg/dose, q5 minutes PRN.
- Product availability and administration:
  - Injectable: 50 mg/mL.
  - Transdermal patches: 12, 25, 50, 75, and 100 mcg/hr.
  - IV pushes slowly over 2–3 minutes, undiluted or diluted in 10 mL NS or D5W; IM/Subcut undiluted. May also be given by Subcut as a continuous infusion.
  - Transdermal patches used for chronic pain with stable opioid requirements, changed q72h.
  - Wean continuous infusions to prevent withdrawal syndrome.
- Onset, peak effect, and duration: See Table 10.1.
- Pharmacokinetics:
  - Quick onset, short duration with intermittent dosing.
  - Highly lipid soluble (prolonged effects with continuous infusion).
- Contraindications: hypersensitivity to fentanyl, opioid naïvety for transdermal patches.
- Significant drug interactions:
  - Other CNS depressant/respiratory depressant medications (i.e., other opioids, benzodiazepines).
  - MAO inhibitors (increased effect of fentanyl).
  - Fentanyl may increase the effects of β-blockers, diltiazem, verapamil, SSRIs, thiazide diuretics.

TABLE 10.1: Pharmacokinetics of fentanyl via different routes

	IV/Intranasal route	IM/Subcut route	Transdermal
Onset	2–5 min	5 min	6 hrs
Peak effect	5 min	30 min	24 hrs
Duration of action	30–60 min	1–2 hrs	72 hrs

- Adverse effects:
  - Excessive sedation.
  - Respiratory depression.
  - Chest wall rigidity (rapid IV administration).
  - Dizziness.
  - Drowsiness.
  - Pruritus.
  - Rash (topical patch).
  - Hypokalemia.
  - Constipation.
  - Urinary retention.
- Monitoring: HR, RR, BP, oxygen saturation, reduction in pain score, and level of sedation.
- Fentanyl special considerations and pearls:
  - Intermittent IV pushes should be administered *slowly* (over 2–3 minutes, if possible) to prevent chest wall rigidity and respiratory depression.
  - Chest wall rigidity/apnea from rapid IV administration may be reversed with neuromuscular blocker. Be prepared to intubate the patient.
  - Respiratory depressant effect may outlast analgesic effect.
  - More lipid soluble than morphine, thus more potent.
  - No histamine release, thus less bradycardia and hypotension than morphine.
  - Increased body heat increases topical absorption of fentanyl from patch.
  - Only certain manufacturer's patches may be cut (matrix vs. reservoir delivery).
  - Atomizing intranasal delivery device preferred for increased tolerability and absorbable surface area (vs. drops to nares).

Hydromorphone

- Synthetic opioid analgesic (increased potency compared to morphine), and antitussive.
- Binds to μ-opioid receptors in the CNS for analgesia, and acts centrally on the medulla for cough suppression.
- Route of administration: PO, IV/IM/Subcut, and PR.
- Dosing:
  - IV/IM/Subcut intermittent doses: 10–20 mcg/kg/dose IV q2h PRN.
  - Continuous IV/Subcut infusion: 20 mcg/kg bolus, then 2–10 mcg/kg/hr infusion, titrated to effect.
  - PO immediate-release tablets, PO liquid, PR: 0.04–0.08 mg/kg/dose q3–4h PRN.
  - Sustained-release products used for chronic pain and dosed based on average daily requirements of immediate-release preparations, usually dosed q12h.
- Product availability and administration:
  - Injectable – 2, 10, 20, 50 mg/mL.

- PO immediate-release tablets – 1, 2, 4, and 8 mg.
- PO liquid – hydromorphone 1 mg/mL.
- PR immediate-release suppository: 3 mg.
- PO sustained-release capsules (q12h, hydromorph contin) – 3, 6, 12, 18, 24, and 30 mg.
- For chronic pain, sustained-release capsules may be opened and sprinkled on food (pellets to be swallowed whole).
- IV pushes undiluted or diluted to 10 mL with NS or D5W over 2 minutes.

- See Table 10.2 for onset, peak effect, and duration.
- Pharmacokinetics:
  - Well absorbed orally, some variability with IM absorption (may have slower onset IM).
  - Metabolized in the liver via glucuronidation to inactive metabolites.
  - Primarily eliminated by the kidneys.
- Contraindications: hypersensitivity to hydromorphone.
- Significant drug interactions:
  - Other CNS depressant/respiratory depressant medications (i.e., other opioids, benzodiazepines).
  - Hydromorphone may increase levels of SSRIs and thiazide diuretics.
  - Succinylcholine, amphetamines, and antipsychotics may increase the levels/ effects of hydromorphone.
  - MAO inhibitors (increased effect of hydromorphone).
- Adverse effects:
  - Excessive sedation.
  - Respiratory depression.
  - Bradycardia.
  - Hypotension.
  - Dizziness.
  - Drowsiness.
  - Elevated intracranial pressure.
  - Pruritus.
  - Constipation.
  - Urinary retention.
  - GI upset (may take PO with food).

TABLE 10.2: Pharmacokinetics of hydromorphone for different routes of administration

	IV/Subcut route	IM	PO/PR	Sustained-release PO
Onset	5 min	15 min	15 min	60 min
Peak effect	10 min	10 min	30–60 min	4 hr
Duration	4 hr	4 hr	4 hr	12 hr

- Monitoring: HR, RR, BP, oxygen saturation, reduction in pain score, level of sedation, and constipation.
- Hydromorphone special considerations and pearls:
  - Better absorbed orally than morphine.
  - Prescribe oral liquids in mg, not mL.

Methadone

- Long-acting opioid, binds to μ-opioid receptor in CNS.
- Similar analgesic potency to morphine, but much longer duration of action and produces less sedation than morphine.
- Antitussive activity, minimal sedation.
- Route of administration: PO.
- Dosing:
  - 0.1–0.2 mg/kg PO q6h PRN.
  - Adjust dose in renal impairment.
- Product availability and administration:
  - PO immediate-release tablets: 1, 5, and 10 mg.
  - PO oral liquid concentrates: 1 and 10 mg/mL.
  - Oral liquids must be dispensed as diluted oral concentrate in juice to prevent use for injection.
- Onset: 30–60 minutes.
- Peak effect: 2–4 hours.
- Duration: 6–8 hours.
- Pharmacokinetics:
  - Well absorbed orally.
  - Highly protein bound.
  - Metabolized in liver by CYP P450 enzymes, and by *N*-demethylation to inactive metabolites.
  - Eliminated by the kidneys.
- Contraindications: prolonged QT interval, hypersensitivity to methadone.
- Significant drug interactions:
  - Caution with medications that also prolong the QT interval (additive effect as methadone can also prolong QT).
  - Azole antifungals, alfuzosin, amphetamines, ciprofloxacin, MAO inhibitors, quinine, SSRIs, and succinylcholine may increase the levels of methadone.
  - Carbamazepine, phenytoin, barbiturates, and protease inhibitors/non-nucleoside reverse transcriptase inhibitors (NNRTIs) may decrease the levels of methadone.
- Adverse effects:
  - Respiratory depression.
  - Bradycardia.
  - Hypotension.
  - Prolongation of QT interval/Torsade de pointes.
  - Dizziness.

- Drowsiness.
- Diaphoresis.
- Constipation.
- Urinary retention.

■ Methadone special considerations and pearls:
- Pain management dosing different than narcotic addiction dosing (q6h PRN vs. q24h, respectively).
- Less sedation than other opioids.
- Can accumulate with chronic use due to high degree of protein binding, thus a decrease in dose or frequency may be required after 5–7 days.
- Potential for medication error with different concentrations of oral liquids, prescribed in mg, not mL.
- There are regulatory requirements for methadone prescription in many jurisdictions.

PCA Opioids

■ Patient-controlled analgesia (PCA) is a method for delivering continuous infusions of opioid analgesics such as morphine, hydromorphone, or fentanyl.

■ PCA allows a set dose of opioid to be administered on-demand to the patient, at a set interval via an infusion pump.

■ Continuous infusion (i.e., mcg/hr) can also be run via a PCA pump, and the rate of the continuous infusion adjusted based on the record of on-demand doses used.

■ PCA is usually via IV or Subcut route.

■ The advantage of PCA is a more stable and patient-specific delivery of pain control.

■ Patients must be assessed for ability to understand and use PCA correctly.

■ PCA syringes are usually prepared by the Pharmacy Department, under laminar flow in a sterile hood and are affixed with high alert labels to indicate for PCA pump use only.

Example of PCA Morphine

■ Morphine: 125 mg/25 mL syringe (5 mg/mL diluted with NS).

■ PCA dose: usually 10–30 mcg/kg/dose.

■ Lockout interval: 6–10 minutes.

■ Maximum limit per 4 hours: ~1,200 mcg/kg/4 hr or as directed by Acute Pain Service.

■ Continuous infusion: 0–30 mcg/kg/hr.

■ Higher doses may be required for chronic use/opioid tolerance (Table 10.3).

Co-analgesics/Adjunctive Agents

■ Co-analgesics or adjunctive agents are medications used along with opioids and non-opioids to control pain.

■ Use of an adjunctive agent may decrease the required dose for an opioid analgesic (opioid-sparing).

TABLE 10.3: Relative potency of opioids and IV:PO conversions

	Medication	Ratio comparison based on standard of morphine 10 mg IM[a]	
		Equipotent Oral Strength[b] (mg)	Equipotent parenteral strength (mg)
Most potent	Fentanyl	N/A	0.1–0.2
	Hydromorphone	4–6	2
	Morphine	20–30	10
	Methadone	Single dose: 20 Chronic use: 2–4	N/A
Least potent	Codeine	200	120

[a]Based on adult data, unknown direct applicability to pediatric population. Refer to usual initial doses for opioid naïve pediatric patients, and use relative ratio of potency to covert between medications or routes of administration.
[b]For immediate-release oral preparations.

- Adjunctive agents are medications that were originally developed for the treatment of another medical condition, but have been found to have analgesic properties as well.
- The major use of adjunctive agents is for the treatment of neuropathic pain.
- Adjunctive agents can be selected based on the nature of pain, or the adverse effects that may actually be beneficial depending on the patient's presentation.
- Adjunctive agents should always be titrated to an effective dose slowly, and then tapered gradually to discontinue.

Amitriptyline
- Amitriptyline is a tricyclic antidepressant medication, which can also be used to control chronic and neuropathic pain.
- TCAs blunt neuropathic pain by inhibiting reuptake of serotonin and norepinephrine in the CNS, blocking conduction in sodium channels, blocking adenosine receptors, and NMDA receptors.
- Routes of administration: PO.
- Dosing:
  - Amitriptyline: 0.1 mg/kg PO QHS, increase as tolerated over 2–3 weeks to 0.5–2 mg/kg PO QHS.
- Product availability and administration:
  - Amitriptyline: 10, 25, 50, and 75 mg tablets.
- Onset: several weeks of consistent dosing and compliance to achieve adequate relief of neuropathic pain, some relief within 7 days.
- Pharmacokinetics:
  - Well absorbed orally.
  - Highly protein bound (non-dialyzable in toxicity).
  - Metabolized in liver to active metabolite, nortriptyline.
  - Excreted primarily by kidneys.

- Contraindications:
  - Hypersensitivity to TCAs.
- Significant drug interactions:
  - Use of MAO inhibitor within 14 days (risk of serotonin syndrome, hypertensive crisis) – contraindicated.
  - Alfuzosin, bupropion, cimetidine, ciprofloxacin, divalproex, duloxetine, lithium, MAO inhibitors, amphetamines, metoclopramide, protease inhibitors, quinine, SSRIs, terbinafine, and valproic acid may *increase* the levels and effects of amitriptyline.
  - Barbiturates, carbamazepine, St. John's wart may *decrease* the levels of amitriptyline.
- Adverse effects:
  - Sedation – tolerance to sedation usually develops within a few weeks.
  - Anticholinergic effects – tolerance to anticholinergic effects usually develops within a few weeks.
  - Anxiety, worsening depression, suicidal ideation.
  - Postural hypotension.
  - Tachycardia.
  - Weight gain.
  - Photosensitivity, rash.
  - Discoloration of the urine (blue-green).
- Monitoring:
  - Decrease in severity of neuropathic pain over several weeks.
  - Mood, suicidal behaviors, or ideation.
- TCA special considerations and pearls:
  - Caution use in pediatric patients with mood disorder, due to potential initial worsening of depression or suicidal ideation.
  - Narrow therapeutic range, thus toxic in overdose.
  - Routine therapeutic drug monitoring not necessary, but levels may be helpful in suspected toxicity.
  - Amitriptyline may be useful if the patient complains of constant burning pain and trouble sleeping (adverse effect of sedation helpful).

Gabapentin and Pregabalin
- Gabapentin and pregabalin are anti-convulsant medications that can be used for chronic and neuropathic pain in pediatrics that is described as "shooting" pain.
- Mechanism of action is not fully understood.
  - Likely binds to undefined neuroreceptors or a carrier protein.
  - Pregabalin may modulate calcium channels involved in neuropathic pain.
- Gabapentin and pregabalin are structurally similar to the inhibitory neurotransmitter, gamma-amminobutyric acid (GABA), although they do not bind to the GABA receptors.
- Route of administration: PO.

- Dosing:
  - Gabapentin:
    - Day 1 : 5 mg/kg/dose PO QHS.
    - Day 2 : 5 mg/kg/dose PO BID.
    - Day 3 : 5 mg/kg/dose PO TID.
    - Titrate to effect.
    - Usual dose 8–35 mg/kg/day divided TID.
  - Pregabalin: optimal dosing is not well defined.
    - May empirically start at 25 mg PO BID, increased by 25 mg/day to a usual maximum of 150 mg PO BID, or 6 mg/kg/day (titrate to lowest effective dose).
    - Adjust dose in renal impairment.
- Product availability and administration:
  - Gabapentin – 100-, 300-, and 400-mg capsules, 600- and 800-mg tablets, 100-mg/mL oral liquid.
  - Pregabalin – 25-, 50-, 75-, 150-, 225- and 300-mg PO capsules.
- Onset: Several weeks of consistent dosing and compliance to achieve adequate relief of neuropathic pain, some relief within 7 days.
- Pharmacokinetics:
  - Rapid oral absorption via facilitated transport proteins.
  - Low protein binding.
  - Not metabolized (no inactive or active metabolites).
  - Excreted in urine and feces.
- Contraindications
  - Hypersensitivity to gabapentin or pregabalin.
- Significant drug interactions:
  - Ketorolac may decrease the levels of gabapentin.
  - Gabapentin may increase the effects of CNS depressants.
- Adverse effects:
  - Peripheral edema.
  - Restlessness, emotional lability, poor concentration.
  - Increased risk of suicidal behavior and ideation.
  - Dizziness.
  - Fatigue.
  - Dry mouth.
  - Weight gain.
  - Pruritus.
  - Constipation.
  - Diplopia.
- Monitoring
  - Decrease in severity of neuropathic pain over several weeks.
  - Suicidal behaviors or ideation.

- Gabapentin and pregabalin special considerations and pearls:
  - Bioavailability decreases with increasing doses (i.e., giving a higher dose does not always result in greater clinical effect – transport proteins for absorption are saturable).
  - Pregabalin may be titrated more rapidly than gabapentin (better tolerability of pregabalin).
  - Gabapentin oral liquid should be refrigerated.
  - Administering with food can increase absorption.
  - Titrate doses slowly, and taper gradually to discontinue.

Baclofen

- Baclofen is a non-paralytic skeletal muscle relaxant used as an adjuvant medication for patients with persistent muscle spasm and related musculoskeletal neuropathic pain.
- Baclofen is an agonist to the GABA inhibitory neurotransmitter receptor, inhibiting afferent neurotransmission and muscle contraction.
- Routes: PO (intrathecal in severe cases).
- Dosing:
  - Titrate slowly to effect.
  - Less than 2 years old: 10–20 mg/day divided q8h, increase dose q3 days in increments of 5–15 mg/day to reach maximum of 40 mg/day.
  - Two to 7 years old: 20–30 mg/day divided q8h, increase dose q3 days in increments of 5–15 mg/day to reach maximum of 60 mg/day.
  - Greater than 8 years old: 30–40 mg/day divided q8h, increase dose q3 days in increments of 5–15 mg/day to reach maximum of 120 mg/day.
- Product availability and administration:
  - PO tablets: 10 and 20 mg.
  - PO compounded suspension 5 or 10 mg/mL (not commercially available), refrigerate.
  - 0.05 mg/mL and 0.5 mg/mL injection for intrathecal use – requires initial test dose, may be used as continuous intrathecal infusion.
  - Administer PO with food.
- Onset – 3–4 days.
- Peak effect – 5–10 days.
- Duration – 8 hours.
- Pharmacokinetics:
  - Rapid oral absorption.
  - Minimally metabolized in the liver (little active or inactive metabolites).
  - Largely excreted in urine and feces.
- Contraindications:
  - Hypersensitivity to baclofen.
- Significant drug interactions
  - Baclofen increases effect of CNS depressants.

- Adverse effects:
  - Hypotension.
  - Chest pain/palpitations.
  - Dizziness.
  - Insomnia.
  - Headache.
  - Slurred speech.
  - Rash, pruritus.
  - Dry mouth.
  - Anorexia.
- Monitoring: decreased muscle rigidity and spasm, tolerance of dose titration.
- Baclofen special considerations and pearls:
  - Abrupt withdrawal may potentiate seizure activity or hallucinations.
  - Be aware of potential for error with multiple compounded oral liquid concentrations (5 and 10 mg/mL).
  - Prescribe oral liquid in mg, not mL.

Topical Anesthetics

LET Gel

- LET gel contains Lidocaine 4%, Epinephrine (1:2,000) 0.1%, Tetracaine 0.5% in a cellulose gel (without cellulose is LET solution, liquid formulation).
- LET is used for anesthesia of lacerations, most commonly lacerations of the face and scalp in pediatric patients.
- Administration: apply 1–3 mL of solution with cotton-tipped applicator around edges and directly into wound.
- Duration to apply/onset of anesthesia: 20–30 minutes.
- Duration of anesthesia: 30 minutes after application complete.
- LET gel special considerations and pearls:
  - Preferred agent for laceration repair over TAC, and less painful than local infiltration of lidocaine: see Chapter 11.
  - Should not be used on mucous membranes or end-arteriolar peripheral extremities (i.e., finger tips, nose tip, penis, ears) due to vasoconstriction with epinephrine.
  - Avoid in patients with hypersensitivity to amide anesthetic agents.
  - Most studies of LET gel for laceration repair are in children greater than 2 years of age.
  - Should be labeled "*not* for injection," refrigerated and protected from light.
  - Not efficacious for intact skin.

TAC

- TAC is a topical anesthetic, containing Tetracaine 0.5%, Epinephrine 0.05%–0.1%, and Cocaine 11.8%.

- TAC is not a preferred agent for topical anesthesia due to expense, concern of toxicity, and regulatory restriction surrounding use and storage of cocaine.
- LET is equally efficacious, with less adverse effects and restrictions.
- Application: apply 2–5 mL directly to wound with cotton or gauze.
- Duration to apply/onset of anesthesia: 10–30 minutes.
- Duration of anesthesia: 30 minutes after application complete.
- TAC special considerations and pearls:
  - Rare severe adverse effects: seizure, CNS stimulation, peripheral vasoconstriction, tachycardia, and MI.
  - Should not be used on mucous membranes or end-arteriolar peripheral extremities (i.e., finger tips, nose tip, penis, ears) due to vasoconstriction with epinephrine.
  - Tetracaine and cocaine are an ester anesthetics (avoid in patients with hypersensitivity to ester anesthetics).
  - Not efficacious for intact skin.

Eutectic Mixture of Local Anesthetics

- Eutectic mixture of local anesthetics (EMLA®) contains 2.5% lidocaine and 2.5% prilocaine.
- As a eutectic mixture, when combined together, lidocaine and prilocaine dissolve into a liquid preparation, and are available commercially formulated as a cream or as a topical patch.
- Used primarily for reducing pain associated with minor procedures such as venipuncture, vaccinations, and superficial skin procedures (i.e., laser treatments, electrolysis, surgical debridement), as well as relief of pruritus.
- Application:
  - Apply a thick layer (1–2 g/10 cm^2) of cream to intact skin, cover with nonadhesive occlusive dressing (i.e., Tegaderm).
  - Apply patch directly on area to be anesthetized.
- Duration to apply/onset of anesthesia: 1–2 hours.
- Duration of anesthesia: 0.5–2 hours after application complete.
- EMLA special considerations and pearls:
  - Not a preferred agent for topical anesthesia in the emergency department due to long onset of action; efficacy depends on duration of application.
  - Should be used only on intact skin.
  - Significant adverse effects such as contact dermatitis and methemoglobinemia (especially if applied to large areas, repeated doses, nonintact skin, or children <3 months of age).
  - Caution with medications that may also induce methemoglobinemia (i.e., sulfonamides).
  - Other adverse effects: blanching, erythema, and edema at site of application.
  - Avoid on mucous membranes.
  - Avoid in patients with hypersensitivity to amide anesthetics.

Tetracaine (Ametop®)

- Topical anesthetic commercially available as cream containing tetracaine 4%.

- Used primarily as topical anesthetic for venipuncture or IV cannulation.
- Application: apply layer of cream (1 g/30 cm^2 – 6 × 5 cm) to intact skin, cover with nonadhesive occlusive dressing (i.e., Tegaderm).
- Duration to apply/onset of anesthesia: 30–45 minutes.
- Duration of anesthesia: 4–6 hours (application may be repeated after 5 hr, not to exceed 2 g/24 hrs for children).
- Tetracaine special considerations and pearls:
  - Avoid in patients with hypersensitivity to ester anesthetics.
  - Not recommended for children less than 1 month of age.
  - Adverse effects: erythema at application site (vasodilation), edema, and pruritus at application site. Rare blistering may occur.

Lidocaine (Maxilene®)

- Topical anesthetic commercially available as cream for topical application containing lidocaine 4% or 5% in a liposomal formulation.
- Cream used primarily as topical anesthetic for venipuncture, relief of pain, and pruritus associated with minor skin irritations (i.e., superficial burns, insect bites, and scrapes).
- Application of cream: rub pea-sized amount into area to be anesthetized for 30 seconds, and then cover with remaining amount of dose in a thin layer. Occlusive nonadhesive dressing may be used, but is not necessary.
  - Age less than 1 year, or weight less than 10 kg = 1 g per site.
  - Age 1–6 years, or weight 10–20 kg = 2 g per site.
  - Age greater than 7 years, or weight greater than 20 kg = 2.5 g per site (1/2 of 5 g tube).
    - ▶ Maximum dosing: may repeat for each procedure as necessary, up to a maximum of three applications per day, spaced by at least 2 hours.
- Duration to apply/onset of anesthesia: 20 minutes.
- Duration of anesthesia: 1 hour after completion of application.
- Lidocaine special considerations and pearls:
  - Do not use in patients with hypersensitivity to amide anesthetics.
  - Produces less vasodilation than Ametop (potentially less erythema), and less vasoconstriction than other topical anesthetics containing epinephrine (i.e., LET and TAC), thus may lead to greater visibility and success for IV starts.
  - Not recommended for children <1 month of age.
  - Only for use on intact skin.

Suggested Reading

Axelrod FB, Berlin D. Pregabalin: a new approach to treatment of the dysautonomic crisis. Pediatrics 2009;124;743–746.

Bedard M, Massicotte A, Prasad S. Ottawa Hospital Parenteral Drug Therapy Manual, 31st ed. Ottawa Hospital, 2010.

Brunton LL, Lazo JS, Parker KL. Goodman & Gilman's the pharmacological basis of therapeutics, 11th ed. New York: McGraw-Hill, 2006.

Chen J, Wong C, Lau E. Morphine for pain relief in children. Pharmacy connection. Ontario College of Pharmacists, 2011.

Cregin R, Rappaport AS, Montagnino G, et al. Improving pain management for pediatric patients undergoing non-urgent painful procedures. Am J Health Syst Pharm 2008;65:723–727.

Duffett M. Pediatric critical care medication handbook. Hamilton, ON: McMaster Children's Hospital, 2010.

Eichenfield LF, Funk A, Fallon-Friedlander S, et al. A clinical study to evaluate the efficacy of ela-max (4% liposomal lidocaine) as compared with eutectic mixture of local anesthetics cream for pain reduction of venipuncture in children. Pedatrics 2002;109:1093–1099.

Jensen B, Regier LD. Rx files drug comparison charts, 7th ed. Saskatoon, SK: Saskatoon Health Region, 2008.

Jovey RD. Managing pain – Canadian healthcare professional's reference. Canadian Pain Society. Toronto, ON: Healthcare & Financial Publishing, Rogers Media, 2002.

Kalant G, Grant DM, Mitchell J. Principles of medical pharmacology, 7th ed. Toronto, ON: Elsevier Canada, 2007.

Keyes PD, Tallon JM, Rizos J. Topical anesthesia: current indications, options and evidence in the repair of uncomplicated lacerations. Can Fam Physician 1998;44:2152–2156.

Kundu S, Achar S. Principles of office anesthesia: Part II. Topical anesthesia. Am Fam Physician 2002;66(1):99–102.

Lau E. Hospital for Sick Children Drug Handbook and Formulary. Toronto, ON: Hospital for Sick Children Drug Information Service, 2009.

Micromedex Healthcare Series (Intranet database) Version 5.1. Greenwood Village, Colo. Thomson Reuters (Healthcare) Inc.

Pediatric Parenteral Drug Administration Monographs. Hamilton, ON: Hamilton Health Sciences Drug Information Service, 2011.

Phelps SJ, Hak EB, Crill CM. Pediatric injectable drugs, 8th ed. Bethesda, MD: American Society of Health Systems Pharmacists, 2007.

Priestley S, Kelly AM, Chow L, et al. Application of topical local anesthetic at triage reduces treatment time for children with lacerations: a randomized controlled trial. Ann Emerg Med 2003;42:1;34–40.

Repchinsky C. Compendium of pharmaceuticals and specialties. Ottawa, ON: Canadian Pharmacists Association, 2011.

Taddio A, Soin HK, Schuh S, et al. Liposomal lidocaine to improve procedural success rates and reduce procedural pain among children: a randomized controlled trial. CMAJ 2005;172(13):1691–1695.

Taketomo CK, Hodding JH, Draus DM. American pharmacists association pediatric dosage handbook, 17th ed. Hudson, OH: Lexi-Comp, 2010.

Vondracek P, Oslejskova H, Kepak T, et al. Efficacy of pregabalin in neuropathic pain in paediatric oncological patients. Eur J Paediatr Neuro 2009;13(4):332–336.

11 Local Anesthetics

Brian Levy and Jonathan Sherbino

Introduction

- Local anesthetics are commonly used in the emergency department (ED) for laceration repair and regional analgesia.
- Inca Indians first used cocaine, derived from *Erythroxylon coca* bushes found in the Andes during cranial trephination.
- Small nerve fibers are more sensitive to local anesthetics, while myelinated fibers are blocked before nonmyelinated fibers.

Biochemistry

- Generic structure of local anesthetic agents.
  - Aromatic ring (lipophilic) – intermediate chain – hydrophilic tail.
- Anesthetic properties determined by:
  - p*K*a – amount of local anesthetic that penetrates through the tissues.
  - Partition coefficient – intrinsic lipid solubility.
  - Degree of protein binding.
  - Type of intermediate chain determines two basic types: the "esters" and the "amides."
    - ▶ Amino-esters:
      - ○ "Esters" include cocaine, procaine, tetracaine, and chloroprocaine.
      - ○ Esters are hydrolyzed by plasma pseudocholinesterase.
    - ▶ Amino-amides:
      - ○ "Amides" include lidocaine, mepivacaine, prilocaine, bupivacaine, and etidocaine.
      - ○ Easy memory trick: amides have the letter "i" occurring twice in the generic name.

Anatomy of Nerves

- Structure of peripheral nerves.
  - Bundles of individual nerve fibers or fasciculi are encased in a longitudinal array of collagen fibers known as the endoneurium.
  - Buried within the endoneurium are the actual nerve fibers comprised of an axon or multiple axons, which may or may not be myelinated.

- Neuron resides within the fasciculi encased in the endoneurium
  - In general, neurons contain dendrite(s), which act as signal collectors that monitor the environment, receive signals from other neurons and feed information to the neuron body.

Physiology

- Neural impulses are conducted by the axon, which conducts signals from the cell body to a synapse.
- In unmyelinated nerve fibers, conduction moves as a "ripple" along the entire surface of the axon.
- Myelin sheath insulates the axon, speeding impulse conduction.
  - Impulses skip from node to node along these myelinated axons, depolarizing the entire intervening axon segments all at once (salutatory conduction).
- Neural transmission is made possible by specialized voltage-gated sodium channels, which contain a pore allowing selective ion movement.

Mechanism of Action of Local Anesthetics

Effect of pKa

- Upon tissue infiltration, the lipid-soluble nonionized portion of anesthetic diffuses through the tissue, ultimately across the lipid bilayer axonal membrane.
- Nerve tissue is lipophilic (up to and including the axons' myelinated sheathes, which are simply fat).
  - The higher the proportion of nonionic molecules, the greater the degree to which the anesthetic can penetrate the tissue.
  - Only the nonionized portion of the anesthetic solution can penetrate nerve tissue through the axon.
- Clinical effect of given dosage also impacted by pH of the tissue into which the anesthetic is infused:
  - When the pH of the solution or tissue containing the anesthetic is *greater than* the drug's pK_a, then a greater proportion of the anesthetic molecules in solution will be in nonionized form. *Hence, the lower the pK_a, the faster the onset of anesthesia.*
  - Nonionized form is more lipophilic, *therefore enhancing neural tissue penetration and speeding onset of action.*
  - Inflamed tissue and abscesses tend to have low pH, which unfavorably impacts local anesthetic penetration.
- Once within the axoplasm, a portion of the drug re-ionizes, and this ionic portion is thought to enter the sodium channels where it slows the movement of sodium ions, thereby preventing the formation/flow of action potentials.

Effect of Intrinsic Lipid Solubility

- Lipid solubility is typically expressed as "partition coefficient."
  - Partition coefficient compares solubility of agent in a nonpolar solvent with solubility in a polar solvent such as water.

- The greater the partition coefficient, the greater the potency, and more rapid the onset.

Effect of Protein Binding
- Duration of blockade determined by intrinsic protein binding of agent.
  - Higher protein binding causes tighter bonding to sodium channel receptors and greater duration of blockade.

Effect of Vasoconstrictors (e.g., Epinephrine)
- Benefits of adding vasoconstrictors include the following:
  - Slows systemic absorption, allowing increased maximum dosages without increased risk of systemic toxicity.
  - By slowing systemic absorption via local decrease of blood flow, duration of action lengthens.
  - Vasoconstrictors reduce local blood flow, promoting hemostasis and improve visualization of field.
  - Epinephrine typically added in concentrations of 1:100,000 or 1:200,000.
    - Epinephrine does not prolong action of bupivacaine.
    - Traditional texts continue to recommend against use of epinephrine in areas of body perfused only by end arterioles:
      - More recent literature review (regarding digital infiltration) refutes this long-standing "prohibition" as "medical mythology."

Effect of Nerve Anatomy
- When local anesthetics infiltrate a peripheral nerve, they diffuse from the outer surface "mantle" of the nerve toward the inner fibers "core."
  - In general, the mantle fibers innervate more proximal structures anatomically, and core fibers innervate more distal structures.
  - Expect faster onset of nerve block more proximally than distal blocking action.

Local Anesthetic Agents
- See Table 11.1.

Short-Duration Agents
- Procaine:
  - Largely replaced by lidocaine due to high incidence of hypersensitivity reactions.
- Chloroprocaine:
  - Most frequent use has been in short-duration epidural anesthesia.
  - Believed to be the least toxic local anesthetic to the central nervous system (CNS) and cardiovascular system.
    - Prior controversy suggesting neurological deficits after large inadvertent subarachnoid injection.

TABLE 11.1: Local anesthetics

Name generic (trade)	Class	Concentration (%)	Maximum dose (with epinephrine)	Onset	Duration (min)
Short acting					
Procaine (Novocaine)	Ester	1–2	7 mg/kg (9 mg/kg)	10–15	20–30 (30–45)
Chloroprocaine (Nesacaine)	Ester	1–2		6–12	15–30 (30)
Moderate acting					
Lidocaine (Xylocaine)	Amide	1–2	4–5 mg/kg (7 mg/kg)	5–15	30–60 (120)
Mepivacaine	Amide	0.5–1	4–5 mg/kg (7 mg/kg)	5–15	45–90 (120)
Prilocaine (Citanest)	Amide	0.5–1	8 mg/kg	15–25	30–90 (120)
Long acting					
Bupivacaine (Marcaine)	Amide	0.25–0.5	2 mg/kg (3 mg/kg)	15–30	120–240 (180–240)
Ropivacaine (Naropin)	Amide	0.2–0.5		1–15	120–240 (180–240)
Topical tetracaine[a] (Pontocaine)	Ester			3–10	30–60

[a]Topical tetracaine has a fast onset of action and duration. Used primarily for rapid ophthalmic and pharyngeal anesthesia.

- ○ Traced to bisulfite preservative no longer contained in current formulations.
- ○ Lumbar spasms reported with preparations of chloroprocaine that contained EDTA, which is no longer part of current formulations.

Moderate-Duration Agents

- Lidocaine:
  - Most multipurpose and versatile of local anesthetics.
    - ▶ Fast onset and relatively short duration make it ubiquitous agent for lacerations, foreign body removal, abscess drainage, lumbar punctures, catheter insertions, and so forth.
  - Variety of concentrations are available from 0.5%–4%, however, 2% is particularly useful when minimal volume is desirable (e.g., fingers).
  - Now restricted for intrathecal use due to concern that even small doses can induce "transient neurologic symptoms" (TNS), which involves onset of pain in the lower extremities from a few hours to 24 hours after apparently uncomplicated administration of spinal anesthesia.
- Mepivacaine:
  - Lower relative incidence of TNS than lidocaine.
  - Alkalinization with bicarbonate, as with lidocaine, may speed its onset of action.
  - Relative contraindication in pregnancy due to slow fetal hepatic metabolism.

- Prilocaine
  - Rapid metabolism and lower acute CNS toxicity relative to lidocaine suggested potential as an infiltrative agent.
  - At doses >600 mg, ortho-toluidine, a metabolite of prilocaine, converts hemoglobin to methemoglobin.
    - ▶ Of particular concern in topical formulations, where dosing for ENT procedures is not strictly adhered to.

Long-Duration Agents
- Bupivacaine:
  - Slow onset, long duration.
  - Structurally similar to mepivacaine with longer duration of action.
  - Typically used at concentrations of 0.5%–0.75% for major nerve conduction blocks.
  - At 0.25% concentration, stronger sensory than motor blockade makes it very useful for local anesthesia.
    - ▶ Well be suited as spinal/epidural agent for obstetrics and postoperative anesthesia.
    - ▶ Has been mixed with faster onset, short-duration agents such as chloroprocaine to increase speed of onset.
      - ○ Doing so appears to considerably shorten the duration of block.
  - Highly cardiotoxic, likely due to high protein binding and lipid solubility.
    - ▶ May cause conduction blocks, activation of reentrant pathways and refractory ventricular arrhythmias including ventricular tachycardia and ventricular fibrillation.
      - ○ Potential to induce refractory cardiac arrest at concentration of 0.75% if inadvertently injected intravenously.
  - Use with epinephrine does not extend duration of block but does reduce plasma uptake.
    - ▶ Recommended for infiltration with bupivacaine in order to provide forewarning of inadvertent intravascular administration.
    - ▶ Include epinephrine as a marker, subject to physician judgment, when infiltrating potentially toxic dosages.
      - ○ Intravascular injection of epinephrine 10–15 µg/mL in adults causes ≥10 beat/min increase in heart rate and/or ≥15 mm Hg increase in systolic blood pressure.
- Ropivacaine:
  - Relatively new agent designed to retain the long-acting properties of bupivacaine with less cardiotoxicity.
    - ▶ Structurally almost identical to bupivacaine with one fewer carbon in its hydrophilic tail.
  - At low concentrations, ropivacaine may provide an even greater ratio of sensory to motor block than bupivacaine.

- Currently, there is ongoing debate regarding comparable safety and relative toxicity of ropivacaine versus bupivacaine in obstetrical labor and intraoperative anesthesia.

Local Anesthetic Infiltration

- Pain during injection is a common complaint.
- Several means to reduce pain during infiltration include:
  - Using a fine needle (27–30 gauge).
  - Distracting patient as you infiltrate.
  - Infiltrate slowly (30 sec/mL) from proximal toward distal direction.
  - Infiltrate inside the wound edge to reduce pain relative to injecting into intact skin.
  - Warm anesthetic solutions (to ~42°C).
  - Alkalinize the solution.
    - Raises anesthetic solution pH.
      - Increases proportion of molecules in nonionic state, therefore:
        - Faster onset
        - Small amount required for conduction blockade
    - Add sodium bicarbonate (44 mEq/50 mL) to lidocaine in a 1:10 ratio (1 mL bicarbonate added to 10 mL lidocaine).
      - Increases rate of degradation at room temperature, decreasing shelf life by 7 days (therefore, make up as you go to avoid this).
      - More lipid-soluble agents such as bupivacaine precipitate easily; hence, use ratio of 1:50 (0.1 mL bicarbonate to 5 mL bupivacaine).

Side Effects/Complications of Local Anesthetics

Local Anesthetic Systemic Toxicity

- Term coined by the American Society of Regional Anesthesia and Pain Medication (ASRA).
- Tends to affect:
  - Females greater than males.
  - Extremes of age: 16% of cases were below 16 years of age and 30% were older than 60.
- Median time from first injection to symptoms: 53 seconds to 60 minutes.
  - Shorter onset thought to be from intravascular injection.

Pathophysiology

- Local anesthetic systemic toxicity (LAST) is thought to be a function of:
  - Patient factors – baseline health, concurrent medications, for example, comorbid cardiac, pulmonary, renal, hepatic, metabolic, and neurologic disease.

- Choice of anesthetic:
  - ▶ Esters are metabolized through plasma pseudocholinesterase and water-soluble metabolite is excreted.
  - ▶ Patients with sensitivity to succinylcholine, taking cholinesterase inhibitors, or those with myasthenia gravis at increased risk from esters.
  - ▶ Cocaine is exception, which is partially hepatically cleared.
  - ▶ Amides are metabolized through the liver, so caution should be used in administering to patients with hepatic or renal compromise.
- Agent:
  - ▶ Greater danger with more lipid-soluble agents (high potency agents, e.g., bupivacaine).
  - ▶ Ninety percent of cases of LAST involved bupivacaine, ropivacaine, and levobupivacaine.
    - ○ Bupivacaine and etidocaine are more cardiotoxic due to high lipid solubility and ability to blockade specific myocardial sodium channels.
    - ○ Bupivacaine carries even greater cardiotoxicity in pregnancy.
    - ○ Epinephrine exacerbates bupivacaine cardiac toxicity.
    - ○ Neonates are at greater risk for bupivacaine toxicity due to lower levels of albumin leaving more free drug in system, and reduced hepatic blood flow allowing amides not to be fully metabolized.
  - ▶ Amount:
    - ○ Rapid infiltration carries greater risk of toxicity than slow infiltration.
    - ○ Application of all topical at once leads to greater toxicity than application in stages or layers.
  - ▶ Location of block:
    - ○ Toxic levels most often induced by inadvertent intravascular administration.
    - ○ Highly vascularized sites more vulnerable (such as for intercostals blocks).
    - ○ Decreasing order of systemic absorption as follows:
      - ➢ Intercostals.
      - ➢ Intratracheal.
      - ➢ Epidural/caudal.
      - ➢ Brachial plexus.
      - ➢ Mucosal.
      - ➢ Distal peripheral nerves.
      - ➢ Subcutaneous.
    - ○ Physician's response to signs and symptoms:
      - ➢ Timeliness of detection by the healthcare provider.
      - ➢ Beware of tachycardia and dysrhythmias from systemic absorption of epinephrine.

Prevention

- Use the lowest *dose* required for the procedure.
- Aspirate with each injection to detect inadvertent intravascular injection.
- Administer incrementally in 3–5-mL aliquots, allowing approximately one circulation cycle (30–45 sec; longer for distal lower extremities) between injections.
    - Patients with a compromised ejection fraction warrant even slower administration to avoid toxic stacking of doses.
- Use ultrasound guidance where large doses will be administered in order to avoid intravascular injection.
- Monitor patients who have required larger doses post-procedure, since toxic reactions may evolve, in particular, when injecting into areas of swollen tissue.

Signs and Symptoms

- Presentation is highly variable – be on guard!

CNS Toxicity

- Patient presentation varies widely, and these occur in only ~20% of cases.
    - Early symptoms include:
        ▶ Lightheadedness.
        ▶ Circumoral numbness.
        ▶ Metallic taste.
        ▶ Agitation.
        ▶ Slurred speech.
    - Late symptoms include:
        ▶ Seizures.
        ▶ CNS depression.
    - Seizures are the most common sign!
    - LAST induced by direct intravascular injection can bypass milder symptoms and proceed direction to seizures with rapid/simultaneous ignition of cardiac sequelae.

Cardiac Toxicity

- Incidence is less common than CNS toxicity.
- Consequence of direct myocardial sodium channel blockade.
    - May manifest as slower PR or QRS intervals.
    - Sodium blockade can trigger reentrant pathways causing VT or ventricular fibrillation.
- Toxicity is potentiated by concomitant hypoxia, hypercarbia, and/or acidosis.
- The effect is dose dependent.
- Early symptoms include:
    - Hypertension.
    - Tachycardia.
    - Ventricular arrhythmias.

- Late symptoms include:
  - Profound decreased contractility.
  - Bradycardia.
  - Hypotension.
  - Asystole.
- Cardiac toxicity may or may not be preceded by seizures or CNS symptoms.
- Bupivacaine and etidocaine are more cardiotoxic due to high lipid solubility and ability to blockade specific myocardial sodium channels.
  - Bupivacaine carries even greater cardiotoxicity:
    - During pregnancy.
    - When used with epinephrine.
  - In neonates due to lower levels of albumin leaving more free drug in system, and reduced hepatic blood flow allowing amides not to be fully metabolized.
- Beware of tachycardia and dysrhythmias from systemic absorption of epinephrine.

Local and Allergic Effects

- True allergies to amides/esters are rare.
  - Reactions more common with ester metabolite para-aminobenzoic acid (PABA).
  - Much less common are reactions to amides, which are likely due to methylparaben that is used as a preservative in amides.
- Systemic toxicity, vasovagal reaction, and systemic absorption of epinephrine are more common.
- True allergic reactions generally involve cutaneous or upper airway signs.
- Prevention:
  - Switch to a preservative-free solution of the opposite class.
    - For example, if the reaction occurs due to esters, consider cardiac lidocaine, which is preservative-free.
    - Other alternatives:
      - Benzyl alcohol with saline or epinephrine.
        - A solution of 0.9% benzyl alcohol with 1:100,000 epinephrine can be made by adding 0.2 mL epinephrine 1:1,000 to a 20-mL vial of normal saline containing benzyl alcohol 0.9%.
        - Small double-blind randomized controlled trial (RCT) found that the above preparation results in significantly less pain than buffered lidocaine, although the duration of action was substantially less.
      - Diphenhydramine.
        - Similar chemical structure similar to local anesthetics, but differs adequately to avoid cross-reactivity.
        - A 0.5% solution can be made by making a 10:1 dilution using nonpreservative containing normal saline with 5% diphenhydramine (i.e., 50 mg/mL).
        - Small double-blind RCT compared 1% lidocaine to 0.5% diphenhydramine for minor laceration repair found that except on

the face 0.5% diphenhydramine provides equivalent analgesia to lidocaine with no increased pain of injection.

➢ At 1% concentration, diphenhydramine has been found to cause increased pain and/or burning on injection.

➢ Disadvantages to diphenhydramine:

○ Tissue sloughing of cutaneous layer has been reported in concentrations of 1% or higher.

○ Vesicle formation, prolonged anesthesia, paresthesias at concentrations of 2–5%.

Treatment of Severe Systemic Symptoms

■ Be prepared for advanced airway management as necessary.

■ Seizures should be promptly aborted with benzodiazepines.

■ Hyperventilation may be effective by transiently reducing $PaCO_2$ causing vasoconstriction with consequent slowing of drug delivery to the brain.

■ Cardiac arrest should be treated according to advanced cardiac life support (ACLS) guidelines with the following modifications:

● Use small initial doses of epinephrine.

● Amiodarone is the preferred agent to treat ventricular arrhythmias.

● Lidocaine or procainamide is *not* recommended.

● Blockers and calcium channel blockers are *not* recommended.

■ Intralipid therapy:

● Early infusion of 20% lipid emulsion may create a "lipid sink" or serve as an energy store for cardiac myocytes.

▶ Dose:

○ Twenty percent lipid emulsion.

○ Initial bolus of 1.5 mL/kg of lean body mass. A second bolus can be considered after 3–5 minutes if necessary.

○ Follow with infusion of 0.25 mL/kg/min continued for 10 minutes following the reestablishment of hemodynamic stability.

➢ In the event of refractory cardiotoxicity, increase infusion rate to 0.5 mL/kg/min.

➢ The current recommended ceiling of lipid emulsion treatment is 8– 10 mL/kg, administered over 30 minutes.

○ NB: Propofol is not considered an advisable alternative because it has its own intrinsic cardiorespiratory toxicity in high doses.

○ In cases of refractory cardiovascular toxicity, consider use of cardiopulmonary bypass until tissue levels of local anesthetics have cleared.

○ Patients with signs of cardiotoxicity should be monitored for at least 12 hours, since toxic local anesthetic effects can persist or recur even posttreatment.

Topical Anesthetics

- Several topical agents are available.
- See Chapter 11 for more details.
- Specific agents

Cocaine

- Available for prescription as cocaine hydrochloride in topical preparations ranging from 2%–10%.
- Rapidly absorbed through mucous membranes; peak plasma level achieved in 15 –60 minutes.
- Applications:
  - Vasoconstrictive – primary current use in ENT applications (e.g., epistaxis).
  - Potent decongestant for swollen mucous membranes.
  - May be used to numb mucosa in preparation for subsequent submucosal infiltration of lidocaine.

Tetracaine, Adrenaline, Cocaine (TAC)

- Consists of 0.5% tetracaine; 0.05% epinephrine, and 11.8% cocaine.
- Onset 10–30 minutes after applying.
- Applications:
  - Nonmucosal skin lacerations, especially to the face and scalp.

Lidocaine, Epinephrine, Tetracaine (LET) Gel or Solution

- Mixture consisting of 4% lidocaine, 0.5% epinephrine, and 0.1% tetracaine.
- Onset 20–30 minutes from application.
- Applications:
  - Nonmucosal skin lacerations to face and scalp.
  - Slightly less effective on extremities.
  - Does not work on intact skin.

Eutectic Mixture of Local Anesthetics

- Made up of 25 mg/mL of lidocaine and 25 mg/mL of prilocaine, plus a thickener, emulsifier and distilled water to adjust pH to 9.4.
- Anesthetizes to 3 mm within 60 minutes and 5 mm within 120 minutes; as a dental preparation, onset is ~2 minutes.
- A study found that 85% of children treated with eutectic mixture of local anesthetics (EMLA) required no further anesthesia for suturing; however, a 90-minute waiting period is required for adequate penetration, which can limit its use.
- Applications:
  - FDA indication is for use on intact, nonmucosal skin.
  - May be used on extremities but not to the palms and soles.

Liposomal 4% or 5% Lidocaine Cream (Maxilene)
- Onset of action in 30 minutes.
- In general requires about 1/2 the time to achieve anesthesia than EMLA cream.
- Applications:
  - Used commonly for pediatric procedures:
    - Venipuncture.
    - Port-a-cath insertion.
    - Peripheral intravenous insertion.
    - Other painful procedures.
  - Temporary relief from minor cuts and abrasions.
  - Penile meatotomy.

Agents for Specific Conditions
- Minor hemorrhoid pain, pruritus ani.
  - Prescription medications:
    - Proctosedyl – hydrocortisone, framycetin sulfate, cinchocaine hydrochloride, aesculin.
      - Available in ointment and suppositories.
        - Anusol-HC 2.5% hydrocortisone with anti-inflammatory, antipruritic, vasoconstrictive properties.
        - RectaGel HC – Lidocaine 2.8% and hydrocortisone acetate 0.55%.
  - Over the counter:
    - Anusol Plus Ointment, suppositories (contain pramoxine).
    - Sandoz Anuzinc Plus.
- Pharyngitis:
  - Benzydamine 0.15% (requires prescription).
    - An indazole nonsteroidal anti-inflammatory drug (NSAID) with analgesic, antipyretic, and anti-edema properties.
      - Unlike other NSAIDs, benzydamine hydrochloride does not inhibit cyclooxygenases (COX) but:
        - Stabilizes membranes, resulting in local anesthesia.
        - Inhibits the production of pro-inflammatory cytokines.
        - Inhibits the generation of reactive oxygen species by neutrophils.
        - Inhibits leukocyte aggregation and adhesion.
        - Exhibits antimicrobial properties.
        - Also used 1 day prior to radiation therapy and continued during treatment to avoid radiation-induced mucositis.
        - Not commercially available in the United States.
        - Not established for use in patients <6 years of age.
        - Gargle or rinse 15–30 seconds, then expel every 1.5–2 hours.
        - Trade names: Apo/Ratio/Dom/Novo/PMS-Benzydamine; Sun-Benz, Tantum.

- Phenol 1.4–1.5% (no prescription required):
  - ▶ Antiseptic/analgesic.
  - ▶ Commercially available as Chloraseptic sprays.

Suggested Reading

Becker DE, Reed KL. Essentials of local anesthetic pharmacology. Anesthesia progress 2006;53:98–109.

Bischof R. Tetracaine, adrenaline, cocaine (TAC) confusion. Pediatrics 1996;97: 287–288.

Crystal CS, Blankenship RB. Local anesthetics and peripheral nerve blocks in the emergency department. Emerg Med Clin North Am 2005;23:477–502.

Crystal CS, McArthur TJ, Harrison B. Anesthetic and procedural sedation techniques for wound management. Emerg Med Clin North Am 2007;25:41–71

Dipchand A, Friedman J, Bismilla Z, et al. The hospital for sick children handbook of pediatrics. Toronto, ON: Saunders Elsevier, 2009.

Dire DJ, Hogan DE. Double-blinded comparison of diphenhydramine versus lidocaine as a local anesthetic. Ann Emerg Med 1993;22:1419–1422.

Eichenfield LF, Funk, A, Fallon-Friedlander S, et al. A clinical study to evaluate the efficacy of ELA-Max (4% liposomal lidocaine) as compared with eutectic mixture of local anesthetics cream for pain reduction of venipuncture in children. Pediatrics 2002;109:1093.

Katis PG. Epinephrine in digital blocks: refuting dogma. CJEM 2003;5(4):245–246.

McGee DL. Anesthetic and analgesic techniques. In: Roberts JR, Hedges JR, eds. Clinical procedures in emergency medicine. Philadelphia, PA: Saunders Elsevier, 2010.

Neal JM, Bernards CM, Butterworth JF, et al. ASRA practice advisory on local anesthetic toxicity. Reg Anesth Pain Med 2010;35(2):152–161.

Scarfone RJ, Jasani M, Gracely EJ. Pain of local anesthetics: rate of administration and buffering. Ann Emerg Med 1998;31:36–40.

Stoelting RK, Miller RD. Basics of anesthesia. Philadelphia, PA: Churchill-Livingstone Elsevier, 2007.

Tetzlaff JE. The pharmacology of local anesthetics. Anesthesiol Clin North America. 2000;18:2:217–233.

Valani R. Pain management and sedation. In: Mikrogianakis A, Valani R, Cheng A, eds. The hospital for sick children manual of pediatric trauma. Philadelphia, PA: Wolters Kluwer/Lippincott Williams & Wilkins, 2008.

Weinberg GL, Ripper R, Murphy P, et al. Lipid infusion accelerates removal of bupivacaine and recovery from bupivacaine toxicity in the isolated rat heart. Reg Anesth Pain Med 2006;31:296–303.

Weinberg GL. Treatment of local anesthetic systemic toxicity. Reg Anesth Pain Med 2010;35:186–191.

Zempsky WT, Karasic RB. EMLA versus TAC for topical anesthesia of extremity wounds in children. Ann Emerg Med 1997;30:163–166.

12 Regional Nerve Blocks

Brian Levy and Jonathan Sherbino

Introduction

- Regional nerve block is a common procedure in the emergency department (ED).
- Can be used for reduction of pain and/or facilitation of painful procedures (e.g., suturing, fracture, or dislocation reduction), especially in anatomical areas, where a large anesthetic field can be achieved distal to the block.
- Advantages of using a nerve block include the following:
  - Allows smaller amounts of local anesthetic to be utilized (in comparison to local infiltration), where a wound involves a broad area in a given nerve distribution (e.g., multiple facial lacerations on ipsilateral side).
  - May avoid tissue distortion caused by local infiltration, particularly in cosmetically significant areas (e.g., the vermillion border of the lip).
  - Avoids wound margin distortion caused by infiltration of large volumes of anesthetic.
  - Avoids the pain and anxiety of multiple injections.
  - May eliminate the need (and attendant risks) for procedural sedation.
- Disadvantages include the following:
  - Requires patient cooperation, especially where efficacy of block depends on patient's ability to detect slight paresthesias.
  - Typically, it is a blind procedure in most EDs (performed without aid of nerve stimulator or ultrasound guidance).
  - Increases risk of anatomical injury (e.g., pneumothorax).
  - Damage to peripheral nerve (1.9 per 10,000).
  - Increases risk of ineffective block (erroneous placement of anesthetic).
  - Risk of systemic toxicity (7.5 per 10,000) from inadvertent intravascular injection.
  - Hematoma.
  - Local infection.
  - Pain at site of injection.

Contraindications

Absolute Contraindications

- Patients suffering from psychosis or dementia, thereby making procedure difficult or patient unable to give informed consent.
- Infection superficial to area of infiltration.
  - Do not inject through infected tissue.
    - ▶ Less effective anesthesia in infected tissue, especially in an abscess due to acidic environment.
    - ▶ Injection into or through infected tissue can induce local or systemic spread of infection.
- Hypersensitivity to local anesthetics – occurs in ~1% of the population.
- Known allergy.
- On anticoagulation (see below).

Relative Contraindications

- Patients unable to communicate during procedure.
  - Severe pain may indicate intraneural injection, which can produce ischemic nerve injury.
- Patient objection to remaining awake.
- Preexisting neuropathy.
- History of malignant hyperthermia.
- Uncontrolled seizure disorders.
- Coagulation disorders or anticoagulation therapy.
  - Absolute contraindication to peripheral nerve blockade when it involves:
    - ▶ Passage of needle deep within muscle mass.
    - ▶ Paravertebral blocks or approaches.
    - ▶ Risk of noncompressible arterial/venous puncture.
    - ▶ Risk of hematoma with subsequent local mass effect on airway.
    - ▶ Postsurgical thromboprophylaxis is not a contraindication to preoperative blockade.

Preparation

- Appropriate history and physical examination, including (but not limited to):
  - Anticoagulant therapy.
  - Sensory or motor deficits, especially in area to be anesthetized.
  - Uncontrolled seizure disorders.
  - Evaluation of distal neurovascular status prior to regional.
    - ▶ Skin color, temperature, capillary refill time, and pulses.
    - ▶ Sensation.
    - ▶ Motor function.
- Explanation of the procedure to the patient.
  - Informed consent should be recorded in the chart.

- Prepare appropriate monitoring and resuscitation equipment to detect and response to possible complications of the procedure.
- Position patient properly.
- Identify and mark landmarks (using ultrasound where possible).
- Antiseptic (e.g., chlorhexidine) skin preparation.
- Surgical draping of the filed field.
- Universal precautions (mask, gloves, eye shields, and contact precautions as indicated).
- Consider placement of intravenous catheter in the event the patient requires supplemental and/or emergency treatment.
- Supplemental:
  - Consider topical premedication of area to be injected to help reduce pain of injection.

General Techniques

- In every procedure, aspirate at each location prior to injection to avoid intravascular injection of the local anesthetic.
- Local infiltration of puncture site with 1% or 2% lidocaine facilitates procedure.
- Inject perineural region not intraneural.
  - Perineural injection may invoke very brief sensory paresthesia indicating anesthetic reaching nerve distribution, however, despite old adage "no paresthesias, no anesthesia" paresthesias may also mark intraneural injection, especially persistent paresthesia during injection.
  - Paresthesias during injection may portend residual neuropathy even if not injected in the intraneural region.
  - Upon encountering paresthesias (prior to infiltration), relocate needle to prevent intraneural injection.
    - ▶ Intraneural injection may cause nerve ischemia and damage via elevated nerve sheath pressure.
    - ▶ May cause prolonged and intense pain.
    - ▶ Immediately terminate injection and reposition needle a few millimeters away, wait for pain to subside, and reinject.
- Three-ring syringe simplifies aspiration, improves control, and eases refilling.
- Choice of agent – see Chapter 11.
- Identifying point of infiltration:
  - ▶ Using anatomical landmarks.
  - ▶ Ultrasonography.
    - ○ Advantages:
      - ➤ Shortens procedural time requirements.
      - ➤ Reduces blind needle passes.
      - ➤ Reduces dosages of anesthetic required to achieve block.
      - ➤ Allows visualization of neighboring structures, for example, pleura, avoiding pneumothorax.

> ➤ Avoid intravascular injection.
> ➤ Accuracy.
- ○ Nerve stimulators:
  - ➤ Not routine practice in most EDs.
- ▪ Maintain high index of suspicion for local anesthetic systemic toxicity (LAST) – see Chapter 11.
  - ● Addition of epinephrine 1:200,000 (5 μg/ml) producing tachycardia may signal clinician of impending systemic toxicity.
  - ● See Chapter 11 for additional details on avoiding, recognizing, and managing LAST.
- ▪ Educate patient on:
  - ● Management of postprocedure pain.
  - ● Identification of wound infection.
  - ● Other complications as appropriate.

Head and Neck Regional Blocks

Supraorbital and Supratrochlear Nerve Block
- ▪ Anatomy and region of sensory coverage (see Figure 12.1).
- ▪ Branch of trigeminal nerve (CN V).
  - ● Originates in midbrain comprised of three branches:
    - ▶ Opthalmic V1.
    - ▶ Maxillary V2.
    - ▶ Mandibular V3.

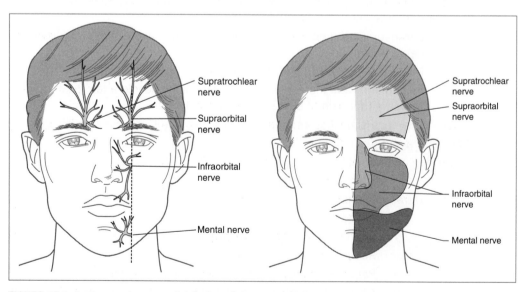

FIGURE 12.1: Anatomy and sensory distribution of the supraorbital, supratrochlear, infraorbital, and mental nerves.

- Supraorbital nerve protrudes through supraorbital foramen directly superior to the pupil and above the superior orbital rim.
- Supratrochlear nerve exits skull just inferior to the orbital rim and 5–10 mm medial to supraorbital foramen.
- Supraorbital nerve supplies most of forehead and supratrochlear supplies ipsilateral surface area of the nose and nasal bridge.
- Forehead supplied by supraorbital and supratrochlear nerves:
  - ▶ Both branch from ophthalmic nerve division (V1) of cranial nerve V (CN V), the trigeminal nerve.
  - ▶ By blocking the supraorbital and infraorbital nerves, complete anesthesia of periorbital area is achieved.
  - ▶ By blocking supraorbital and supratrochlear nerves bilaterally, entire forehead is anesthetized from vertex of scalp to bridge of nose.
- Applications:
  - Wound repair, soft tissue exploration.
- Approach (see Figure 12.2).

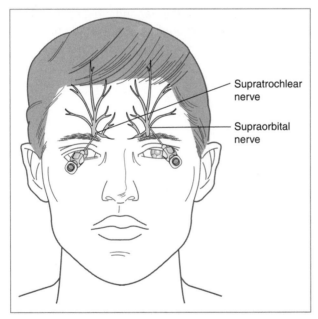

FIGURE 12.2: Approach to supraorbital and supratrochlear nerve block.

Auriculotemporal Block
- External ear and surrounding tissue is innervated by:
  - Auriculotemporal nerve anterosuperiorly and anteromedially extending to more lateral regions of the cheek and temple.
  - Greater auricular nerve, innervating inferoposterior aspects.
  - Minor occipital nerve innervating posterior auricular surface and surrounding tissue.

- Auricular branch of vagus (Alderman's nerve and Arnold's nerve) innervates concha, external auditory canal, and most areas immediately surrounding auditory meatus.
- Applications:
  - Suture of large laceration of ear or surrounding tissue.
  - Excision and drainage of hematoma in area.
- Approach (see Figure 12.3):
  - Prepare ear and surrounding tissue with antiseptic.
  - Infiltrate a track surround the entire ear.
    - ▶ Spirating, infiltrating 3–5 mL of anesthetic as the needle is withdrawing.
    - ▶ Before needle is entirely withdrawn, reorient the needle, fully inserting it just anterior to the ear. After aspirating, infiltrate an additional 3–5 mL along an anterior track as the needle is withdrawn.
    - ▶ Next, introduce the needle just below the earlobe in the sulcus, and repeat the above procedure anteriorly and posteriorly, thus creating another "V"-shaped tract of anesthetic.
- Maximum anesthesia occurs within about 10–15 minutes.
- The superficial temporal artery is medial to the ear and crosses the zygomatic arch. Aspirate to ensure that it is not punctured prior to infiltration.

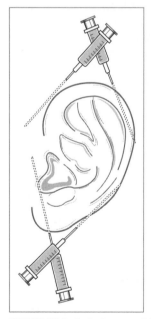

FIGURE 12.3: Auricular nerve block.

Infraorbital Block

- Anatomy (see Figure 12.1):
  - Division of maxillary nerve, V2 of the trigeminal nerve.
  - Exits infraorbital foramen 5–10 mm inferior to the orbital rim and superior but sagittally aligned to the maxillary canine teeth (tooth 6 on the patient's right and tooth 11 on the patient's left).

- Applications:
  - Anesthetizes medial cheek from the lower eyelid running caudally to include the ipsilateral upper lip, and including the medial cheek running laterally to a line drawn vertically at the lateral canthus of the ipsilateral eye.
  - Nasal bridge and nasal folds are generally not part of the geography anesthetized in this approach.
  - Wound closure.
  - Pain relief.
  - Debridement.
- Approach:
  - Intraoral:
    - Position patient supine or sitting.
    - If possible, provide topical anesthesia with a cotton-tipped applicator applied to the oral mucosa superior to the maxillary canines, then dry and retract the upper lip.
    - Stabilize and position the upper lip.
    - Inject at the gingival reflection with the needle at the maxillary canine (tooth 6 or 11) and track superiorly to a point approximately halfway between the entry site and the orbital rim (i.e., this should be just inferior to the infraorbital foramen), and inject 3–5 mL of anesthetic.
      - The anesthetic should be injected adjacent to but not directly into the infraorbital foramen.
      - Direct injection into the foramen may result in swelling of the lower eyelid or possible intraneural injection.
  - Alternative intraoral approach (see Figure 12.4):
    - If uncertain of landmarks or the block is not successful, infiltrate ~5 mL of anesthetic solution intraorally in a fanlike pattern within the upper buccal margin.
      - While lacking precision of a single-targeted injection, a 10–15-second massage of the tissues immediately subsequent to the injection is likely to yield similar anesthesia.

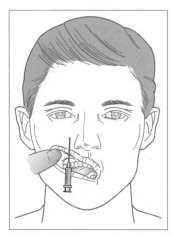

FIGURE 12.4: Approach to infraorbital nerve block (intraoral approach).

- Extraoral:
  - Needle passes closely to facial artery and vein.
    - Do not use vasoconstrictors.
    - Crucial to aspirate before injecting anesthetic.
  - Landmark the infraorbital foramen.
  - Prepare skin in sterile fashion.
  - Advance the needle through the skin, subcutaneous tissue, and quadratus labii superioris muscle.
  - Inject the anesthetic (2–3 mL); infiltrated tissue will swell.
  - Massage the area for 10–15 seconds.

Inferior Alveolar Block and Intraoral Mandibular Block

- Anatomy:
  - Mandibular division of trigeminal nerve (V3) gives rise to:
    - Inferior alveolar nerve
      - Gives rise to mental nerve.
      - Innervates pulp of mandibular teeth from third molar to central incisor.
    - Buccal nerve.
    - Auriculotemporal nerve.
- Applications:
  - Anesthetizes all teeth on ipsilateral side of mandible.
  - Anesthetizes the body of the mandible and the lower portion of the mandibular ramus.
  - Floor of the mouth and anterior two-thirds of the tongue.
  - Anesthetizes anterior mandibular periodontium and lower lip and chin by blocking mental nerve.
- Useful in:
  - Provision of anesthesia for multiple mandibular teeth in anesthetized quadrant and anterior two-thirds of tongue and lingual soft tissues.
  - Patients with dentoalveolar trauma.
  - Postextraction pain.
  - Dry socket.
  - Pulpitis.
  - Abscess.
- Approach (see Figure 12.5):
  - Patient should be seated in a chair with back (such as dental chair or ophthalmic room chair) with occiput firmly against neck support.
  - Apply topical anesthetic if available.
  - Patients are anxious of dental blocks; patient may unexpectedly jerk on contact of needle.
    - Procedure is easiest to achieve with a long needle (minimum 10-mL syringe permits adequate length for direct infiltration), preferably 1⅝ in., 25 gauge, although 1⅛ in., 27 gauge may be even more comfortable for patient.

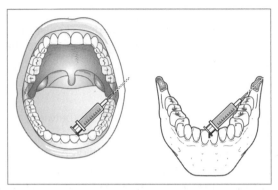

FIGURE 12.5: Approach to inferior alveolar nerve block.

- Palpate the retromolar mandibular fornix with the nondominant gloved thumb to identify the anterior border of the ramus of the mandible; the nondominant index finger should be positioned just anterior to the ear.
- *The mucosa should be stretched* to maximize visibility and reduce pain of injection.
- Specifically, note the *coronoid notch,* which is the greatest concavity on the anterior border of the ramus of the mandible.
  - ▶ Inject at the *height* of this deepest concavity of the ridge.
  - ▶ Move thumb medially from the coronoid notch to palpate the next prominence medially, which is known as the *internal oblique ridge.* The needle will be inserted just medial to the internal oblique ridge at the deepest height of the notch.
  - ▶ Inject 1.5–2 mL of anesthetic. If analgesia is not achieved, two more similar injections may be made.
    - ○ Delayed trismus and sensory deficit have been reported.

Mental Nerve Block
- Anatomy (see Figure 12.1):
  - Mental nerve is terminal sensory branch of inferior alveolar nerve exiting mandible through mental foramen.
  - The mental foramen is in-line with the pupil and generally lies midway between the alveoli (tooth sockets) and the inferior border of the mandible.
  - Innervates lower lip and chin.
  - Three branches:
    - ▶ One branch supplies skin of chin.
    - ▶ The other two branches innervate skin and mucous membrane of lower lip.
- Applications:
  - Provides anesthesia for repair of lacerations of the lower lip or chin.
  - Does not provide anesthesia for teeth, tongue, vestibule, or other soft tissue of the oral mucosa.
  - Easier to perform and less painful than other intraoral blocks.

- Approach (see Figure 12.6):
  - Patient should be seated in chair with back (such as dental chair or ophthalmic room chair) with occiput firmly against neck support so that when mouth is open mandible is parallel to the floor.
  - Locate mental foramen.
    - ▶ Mental foramen should be located:
      - ○ Between teeth 21 and 22 or between 27 and 28 (between canines and first premolars in adults).
      - ○ Between first and second primary molars in children.
  - Needle should be inserted into the gingival reflection between the subject teeth, injecting approximately 2–4 mL of anesthetic solution *near, but not into the mental foramen.*
    - ▶ Injecting into the foramen can cause permanent damage to the neurovascular bundle.

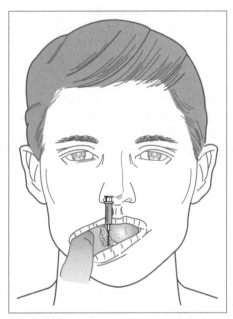

FIGURE 12.6: Approach to mental nerve block.

Superior Alveolar Block

- Anatomy:
  - Division of V2, maxillary division of trigeminal nerve (CN V) further divided into:
    - ▶ Anterior superior alveolar (ASA):
      - ○ Branches from maxillary nerve immediately proximal to its exit from infraorbital foramen.
      - ○ Supplies upper incisor and canine teeth.
    - ▶ Middle superior alveolar (MSA):
      - ○ Branches from infraorbital portion of maxillary nerve.
      - ○ Innervates maxillary premolars (bicuspids) and part of first molar roots.

▶ Posterior superior alveolar (PSA):

   ○ Branches from maxillary nerve just proximal to infraorbital groove.

   ○ Innervates second and third maxillary (upper) molars and two of the three roots of the first maxillary molars.

● Lingual gingiva is *not* innervated by superior alveolar and this block will *not* anesthetize palatine structures.

■ Applications:

● Anesthesia of branches associated with trauma or dental pain to teeth innervated by respective branches of ASA, MSA, or PSA.

● Dentoalveolar abscesses.

● Postextraction and dry socket pain.

■ Approach (see Figure 12.7):

● Patient should be seated in chair with back (such as dental chair or ophthalmic room chair) with occiput firmly against neck support so that when mouth is open mandible parallel to floor.

● ASA nerve block:

   ▶ Retract the lip exposing the mucobuccal fold where it joins the apex of the canine tooth.

   ▶ With the lip retracted, insert needle into the intersection of the mucobuccal fold and the canine at an angle of 45 degree, and advance the needle about 1–1.5 cm.

   ▶ Slowly inject 2 mL of local agent; massage for 10–20 seconds.

● MSA nerve block:

   ▶ Retract the lip exposing the mucobuccal fold where it intersects the joint of the maxillary premolar 2 and molar 1 (teeth 3 and 4, or teeth 13 and 14 in an adult).

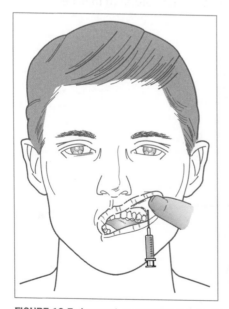

FIGURE 12.7: Approach to superior alveolar block.

▶ With the lip retracted, insert needle into the intersection of the mucobuccal fold and these two teeth at an angle of 45 degree, and advance the needle about 1–1.5 cm.

▶ Slowly inject 2–3 mL of local agent; massage for 10–20 seconds.

● PSA nerve block:

▶ Retract the lip exposing the mucobuccal fold where it intersects the joint of the maxillary molars 1 and 2 (teeth 2 and 3, or teeth 14 and 15 in an adult).

▶ With the lip retracted, insert needle into the intersection of the mucobuccal fold and these two teeth at an angle of 45 degree, and then advance it toward the posterolateral maxillary tuberosity (up, back, and inward) along the natural curve of the maxilla to a depth of 2–2.5 cm.

▶ If the needle hits the bone, withdraw slightly and redirect more laterally.

▶ Slowly inject 2–3 mL of local agent; massage for 10–20 seconds.

Blocks of the Trunk

Intercostal Nerve Block (ICNB)

◾ Anatomy (see Figure 12.8):

● Each intercostal block provides anesthesia to the nerve running above and below a given rib.

● Vein, artery, nerve (VAN) arranged run from superior to inferior within the costal groove at the inferior end of each rib.

● Ribs 1–6 obscured by rhomboids and scapular position making blocks difficult.

● Whether fracture anterior or posterior, it is best to block at "rib angle" just lateral to paraspinal muscles, or ~6 cm lateral to midline.

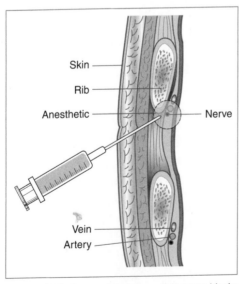

Skin
Rib
Anesthetic — Nerve

Vein
Artery

FIGURE 12.8: Approach to intercostals nerve blocks.

- By blocking posterior to the midaxillary line both divisions of the intercostal nerve, lateral pectoral cutaneous branch and anterior pectoral cutaneous branch are blocked.
- Indications:
  - Relief of posttraumatic pain, postoperative, or postinfectious pain emanating directly from thoracic or abdominal walls.
  - Partial or complete substitute for opiates in cases of severe pain involving:
    ▶ Rib fractures:
      ○ Immediately relieves pain and improves pulmonary mechanics.
      ○ Improves mobility.
    ▶ Dislocation of costochondral joints.
    ▶ Herpes zoster.
    ▶ Nerve entrapment within the rectus abdominis.
    ▶ Blockade at the posterior axillary line provides relief from somatic pain but not visceral pain from thoracic or abdominal organs.
- Approach (see Figure 12.8):
  - Intercostal nerves must be blocked proximal (posterior) to fracture site.
  - Overlapping innervation from segments above and below dictates that *the nerves above and below fractured rib(s) must be blocked.*
  - Nondominant index finger hand palpates the inferior intercostal space and shift skin and subcutaneous tissue cephalad until the inferior edge of the rib is appreciated.
  - This technique allows nondominant index finger to serve as guide and help protect against pneumothorax while helping to ensure optimal block.
  - Insert needle angled cephalad approximately 10–15 degrees, using nondominant index finger as a guide.
  - Penetrate skin and raise subcutaneous wheal and wait 5–10 seconds for anesthesia, then advance until needle contacts bone.
  - Retracted skin is then released by nondominant hand, and needle is walked caudally *very gently* until it falls off inferior edge of rib.
  - Needle then advanced ~3 mm, which is at the costal groove.
  - *Aspirate to ensure neither blood nor air* (e.g., pneumothorax) is returned, then deposit 2–5 mL of anesthetic.
  - Patient should be observed for signs of systemic toxicity or pneumothorax (e.g., hypoxia, shortness of breath or cough) for 30 minutes.
    ▶ Consider chest x-ray in debilitated patient or if in doubt.
    ▶ Three-year retrospective chart study of 160 trauma patients indicates incidence of an individual block causing pneumothorax about 1.4% per individual intercostal nerve blocked.
- Complications:
  - Bilateral intercostal blocks could impair respiration.
  - Pneumothorax.
  - Instances of multiple fractures and multiple blocks introduce potential for local anesthetic toxicity.

Upper Extremity Blocks

Wrist Block

- Anatomy (see Figure 12.9):
  - Ulnar nerve:
    - Originates from the medial cord of brachial plexus.
    - Becomes superficial in distal forearm bound by fascia to the *anterior surface* of flexor retinaculum and carpal tunnel.
    - Travels across wrist joint passing above ulnar styloid with ulnar artery.
    - Innervation of flexor pollicis brevis, abductor pollicis, palmaris brevis, hypothenar muscles (abductor digiti minimi, flexor digiti minimi, and opponens digiti minimi), medial two lumbricals, and all interosseous muscles.
      - Sensation generally to hypothenar surface, dorsal medial surface of palm, medial wrist, fifth digit, and medial half of fourth digit.
  - Median nerve:
    - Arises from parts of the medial and lateral cords of the brachial plexus.
    - Median nerve trunk passes deep to flexor retinaculum into the carpal tunnel.
    - NB: palmar branch of median nerve crosses superficial to flexor retinaculum and remains unaffected by carpal tunnel syndrome.
    - Motor control of thenar muscles (abductor pollicis brevis, flexor pollicis brevis, and opponens pollicis) and first, second lumbricals.
    - Sandwiched in the middle of the wrist between large tendons of palmaris longus and flexor carpi radialis (the prominent tendons on wrist flexion) at proximal wrist crease.
  - Radial nerve:
    - Largest terminal branch of posterior cord of brachial plexus.
    - Divides into superficial and deep branches at antecubital fossa.
    - No motor control of hand muscles.
    - Sensory fibers innervate lateral aspect of wrist and dorsolateral aspects of hand.

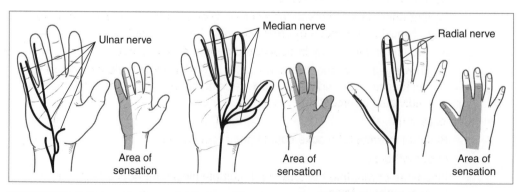

FIGURE 12.9: Anatomy and sensory distribution of the ulnar, median and radial nerves.

- Indications:
  - Anesthesia, depending on nerves blocked for aspects of hands, wrists, and digits for facilitation of wound repair, casting, splinting, or hand surgeries.
  - Entrapment neuropathies.
- Blocking all of the nerves below will anesthetize the entire hand, with the exception of a 2–3-cm patch on the volar aspect of the thenar eminence at the base of the thumb innervated by lateral antebrachial cutaneous nerve.
  - Anesthesia to this area may be provided by infiltrating a wheal just proximal to this area – proximal to the flexor crease of the wrist.
- Approach:
  - Document neurovascular status before beginning the procedure.
  - Prepare sterile site 1–2 cm proximal to the medial distal wrist crease.
  - Hand and wrist in supine position.

Radial Sensory Fibers

- On the dorsal surface, raise a wheal above the radial styloid (3–5 mL of local anesthetic) and infiltrate a subcutaneous tract as shown in Figure 12.10. Fan out in order to create a field block anesthetizing the sensory branches of the radial nerve with another 3–5 mL of local anesthesia.

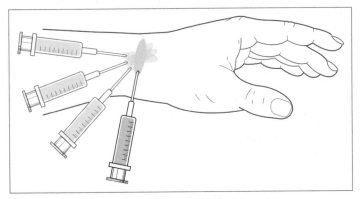

FIGURE 12.10: Infiltration for radial nerve block at the wrist.

Median Nerve

- Through the volar surface, insert the needle about 1 cm ulnar to the palmaris longus (see Figure 12.11).
- Continue to advance the needle until a "pop" is felt as flexor retinaculum is penetrated, then inject 3–5 mL of anesthetic agent.
- If no pop is perceived and bone is contacted, withdraw the needle 2–3 mm, and inject the anesthetic.
- To increase block efficacy, withdraw needle to level of skin, redirect needle laterally 30 degrees and again medially 30 degrees and reinsert, infiltrating 1–2 mL of additional anesthetic in each of these two directions.

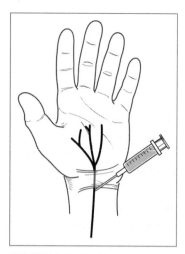

FIGURE 12.11: Median nerve block at the wrist.

Ulnar Nerve

■ Along the ulnar aspect of the wrist, insert the needle just under the flexor carpi ulnaris tendon (see Figure 12.12).

■ Advance needle to a depth of 1.5 cm, after aspiration, inject 5–7 mL of anesthetic solution.

   ● Ulnar artery is immediately lateral to ulnar nerve; achieve negative aspiration before injecting.

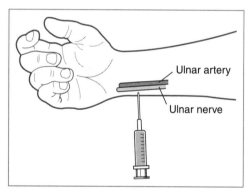

FIGURE 12.12: Ulnar nerve block at the wrist.

Digital Blocks

■ Anatomy (see Figure 12.13):

   ● Volar digital nerves emanate from median and ulnar nerves, while the dorsal digital nerves emanate from radial and ulnar nerves.

   ● Nerves course along both dorsal and ventral sides along each of the phalanges and on both medial and lateral sides.

■ Indications:

   ● Laceration repair.

   ● Drainage of paronychia.

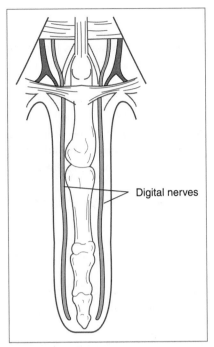

FIGURE 12.13: Anatomy of the digital nerve.

- Fracture or dislocation reduction.
- Nail removal and nail bed repair.
■ Documentation – note neurovascular status prior to block.
  - Capillary refill.
  - Two point discrimination (2–4 mm on volar pads; compare contralateral side).
  - Motor function.
  - Integrity of tendons.
■ Approaches (see Figure 12.14):

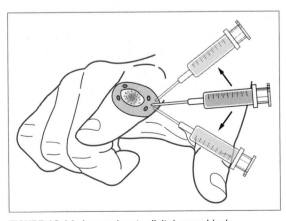

FIGURE 12.14: Approaches to digital nerve block.

- Ring block:
  - ▶ Hand and finger in prone position.
  - ▶ Insert needle into dorsal aspect of webspace at 45 degrees just distal to metacarpophalangeal (MCP) joint at the level where skin texture changes and advance needle toward volar end of the bone.
  - ▶ As bone is gently contacted, withdraw the needle 3–4 mm, aspirate, and then deposit 2 mL of anesthetic in a volar direction.
  - ▶ Withdraw and readvance needle to the dorsal aspect of the phalanx just distal to the MCP joint, aspirate, and then deposit an additional 1 mL.
  - ▶ Withdraw the needle, and repeat the procedure on the opposite side of the finger.
  - ▶ In order to achieve sufficient anesthesia wait for 10–15 minutes before commencing procedure.
- Transthecal/digital sheath (volar) block:
  - Requires only one injection but provides anesthesia to both volar and dorsal surfaces.
    - ▶ Does not anesthetize proximal dorsal surface to level of DIP joint.
    - ▶ Typically requires only 1.5–3 mL of anesthetic to block entire finger versus approximately double that in a classic ring block.
    - ▶ Relatively less risk of trauma to neurovascular bundles than classic ring block.
  - Deposit anesthetic into the flexor tendon sheath in order to anesthetize the digital nerves.
  - Approach:
    - ▶ Inject just distal to the MCP joint (slightly proximal to the first digital crease).
    - ▶ Insert needle at an angle of 90 degrees to proximal digital crease *in the midline of the digit,* avoiding neurovascular bundles.
      - ○ Needle should penetrate skin, subcutaneous tissue, tendon sheath, and the flexor tendon.
      - ○ Advance the needle until bone is gently contacted.
      - ○ Withdraw needle 2–3 mm, leaving the tip of the needle within the flexor tendon sheath.
      - ○ Expect little or no resistance initially; infiltrate 1.5–3 mL of anesthetic solution; expect increasing resistance and possible slight flexion as the sheath fills.
      - ○ Patient should experience digital anesthesia within 2–3 minutes.
- Complications:
  - Ischemia.
  - Neuropathy, intraneural injection.

Lower Extremity Blocks

Femoral Nerve Block
- Anatomy (see Figure 12.15):

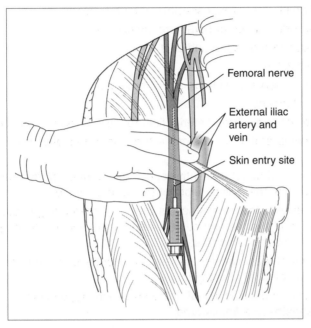

FIGURE 12.15: Approach to femoral nerve block (FNB).

- Femoral nerve is the largest terminal branch of lumbar plexus, comprised of dorsal divisions of anterior rami of L2–L4.
- Courses through psoas muscle, leaving psoas at its lateral border, and then descending into the thigh in the groove between psoas and iliacus muscles, coursing beneath the inguinal ligament.
- A few centimeters below the inguinal ligament, femoral nerve divides into anterior and posterior branches.
  - At this level, the femoral nerve is just lateral and slightly posterior to the femoral artery.
  - After dividing into anterior and posterior branches:
    - Anterior branch of femoral nerve:
      - Supplies motor innervation to the sartorius and pectineus muscles.
      - Provides sensation to skin of anterior and medial thigh.
    - Posterior branch of the femoral nerve.
      - Supplies motor innervation to the quadriceps.
      - Sensory innervation to the medial aspect of the lower leg (saphenous nerve).
- Indications:
  - Anesthesia to anterior thigh and medial leg.
    - Reliable block to femoral and lateral femoral cutaneous nerves; inconsistently blocks obturator nerve.

- Proximal femur and hip fractures, especially in elderly people.
  - ▶ May allow for reduced use of parenteral analgesia.
- Analgesia for procedures on knee and thigh.
- Approach (see Figure 12.15):
  - Use of ultrasound or nerve stimulator is recommended.
  - Identify the femoral artery.
  - Mark the site and prepare a broad sterile field to include the inguinal crease.
  - Raise a wheal 1 cm lateral to the femoral artery and at the level of the inguinal crease.
  - Advance the needle and direct it slightly cephalad, stopping approximately 2–3 cm below the skin, the typical depth of the femoral nerve.
    - ▶ If the patient experiences paresthesias over the anterior thigh caused by the activation of the femoral nerve, withdraw the needle slightly just enough for the paresthesias to stop.
  - Inject 5 mL aliquots of local anesthesia, aspirating between each injection, to a total of 20–30 mL of local anesthetic.
  - Typical time to onset of block is 10–30 minutes depending on type and dosage of local anesthetic administered.

"Three-in-One" Block

- Used to improve performance of femoral nerve block (FNB) especially in relieving pain sensation from the obturator nerve.
- Indication:
  - To anesthetize the femoral, obturator, and lateral femoral cutaneous nerves in patients with hip fractures.
  - Anesthesia of obturator nerve, in particular, may be weak in the typical FNB described above.
  - The obturator nerve receives sensory impulses from the medial aspect of the thigh and provides motor innervation of the adductor muscles.
- Approach:
  - Blockade performed in the same manner as FNB described above (Figure 12.15).
  - Prior to infiltration, the hand compresses the area just caudad to the needle to promote cephalad spread of the local anesthetic.
  - Pressure distal to the injection site continues for a total of 5 minutes during and/or after the injection is made.
  - This achieves blockade of all three nerves: the femoral, the lateral femoral cutaneous, and the obturator.
  - The use of ultrasound provides better technique.

Ankle and Foot Blocks

- Anatomy (see Figure 12.16):
  - Remember the "s" implies SENSORY.
    - ▶ Superficial peroneal, Saphenous, and Sural are 100% Sensory

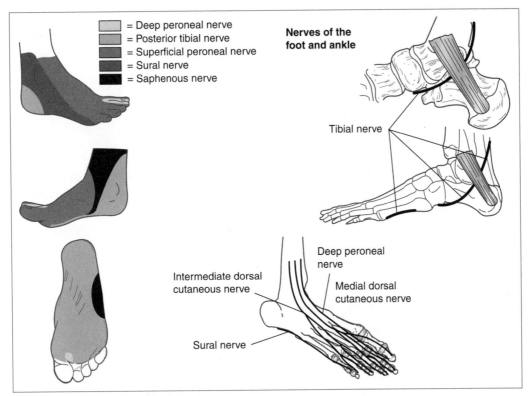

FIGURE 12.16: Innervation of the foot.

- Complete block of sensation and motor innervation of the foot can be achieved by blocking five nerves, all of which originate with the sciatic nerve:
  - ▶ Posterior tibial nerve:
    - ○ Divides into lateral and medial plantar nerves, calcaneal sensory branches, and nerve to the abductor digiti quinti.
    - ○ Provides motor innervation to muscles on plantar side of foot, and sensory innervation over plantar surfaces.
  - ▶ Superficial peroneal nerve:
    - ○ Branch of common peroneal nerve.
    - ○ Purely sensory.
    - ○ Sensory innervation only to dorsal surface of the foot, lateral great toe, and toes two to four.
  - ▶ Deep peroneal nerve:
    - ○ Lateral branch innervates extensor digitorum brevis and extensor hallucis brevis.
    - ○ Sensory innervation to the first web space.
    - ○ Damage including from lateral injury to knee may result in foot drop.

▶ Sural nerve:
  ○ Branch of combined peroneal nerve (anastomotic branch) and tibial nerve (median sural nerve).
  ○ Purely sensory.
  ○ Sensory innervation to dorsolateral surface of foot, including toes four and five.
▶ Saphenous nerve:
  ○ A terminal branch of the femoral nerve.
  ○ Purely sensory.
  ○ Located approximately 1–2 cm anterior to medial malleolus at the ankle.
  ○ Sensory innervation of medial aspect of ankle, foot, and great toe.
■ Applications/indications:
  ● Laceration or wound exploration or repair.
  ● Manipulation of dislocated ankles.
  ● Incision and drainage of abscesses.
  ● Toenail repair.
  ● Fracture reduction.
■ Approach:
  ● Document neurovascular status before and immediately after block.
  ● When administering multiple blocks, block posterior tibial nerve first, since it is the largest.
  ● Ideally, the patient should be supine, with ankle supported by pillow or rolled sheet.

Posterial Tibial Block
  ● Nerve lies in the flexor retinaculum (tarsal tunnel), approximately 1–2 cm posterior to medial malleolus (see Figure 12.17).

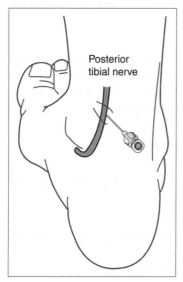

FIGURE 12.17: Posterior tibial nerve block.

- Palpate posterior tibial pulse and inject to its posterior, aspirating to ensure against intravascular injection.
- Inject 5–7 mL, simultaneously palpating to ensure that tendon sheath is filling with anesthetic.
- Wait at least 1–2 minutes before commencing other blocks to discern signs of systemic toxicity or hypersensitivity.
- By waiting 10 minutes, at least partial anesthesia of the foot may be achieved, potentially reducing the pain of other blocks due to overlap of sensory fields.

Deep Peroneal (Fibular) Nerve Block
- Palpate the dorsal pedis pulse (see Figure 12.18).
  - Dorsal pedis pulse is located between the extensor hallucis longus and the extensor digitorum longus.
- Deep peroneal nerve lies lateral to the dorsal pedis pulse.
- Needle should penetrate the skin perpendicularly and advance to the level of the tarsal bones.
- Slowly inject 5–7 mL of local anesthetic.

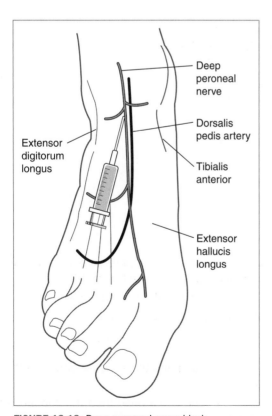

FIGURE 12.18: Deep peroneal nerve block.

Superficial Peroneal Nerve

- Note the broad distribution of sensory fibers across the anterior ankle, in addition to the lateral branch, which is appreciated by plantar flexing the foot and the fourth toe (see Figure 12.19).
- Anesthesia is accomplished *by subcutaneous infiltrations forming a ring between the malleoli*, with a total of 5–10 mL of local anesthetic.

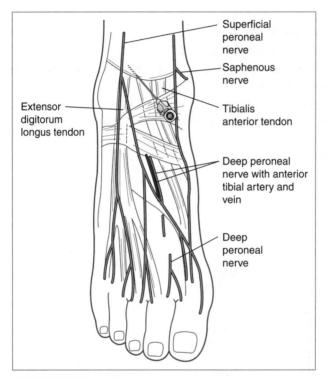

FIGURE 12.19: Superficial peroneal nerve block.

Saphenous Nerve

- Saphenous nerve courses subcutaneously along the anteromedial ankle between the tibialis anterior tendon and medial malleolus (see Figure 12.20).
- Positioned ~2 cm superior and 1 cm anterior to the medial malleolus.
- Inject along this line subcutaneously, approximately 5–7 mL.

Sural Nerve Block

- Identify the area between the Achilles tendon and the superior border of the lateral malleolus (see Figure 12.21).
- After aspirating, inject 5–6 mL of anesthetic into a band from the superior aspect of the malleolus to the Achilles tendon.

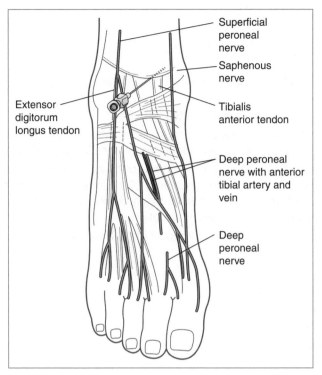

FIGURE 12.20: Saphenous nerve block.

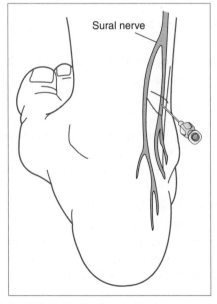

FIGURE 12.21: Sural nerve block.

Other Blocks

Bier Block (Intravenous Regional Anesthesia)

- Indications:
  - Alternative to general anesthesia for short procedures involving upper and lower limbs.
    - Maximum safe duration is 60 minutes.
  - Consider for large lacerations, fracture, or dislocation reductions of forearm, wrist, hand, and other procedures on upper or lower extremities lasting <60 minutes.
    - Used by Farrell et al., safely in children as young as 2 years and elderly patients as old as 86 years by emergency physicians administering 1.5 mg/kg (administered as 0.5% = 5 mg/mL) "mini-dose" of lidocaine for upper extremity fractures and dislocations.
- In all cases, full neurological function returned within 10 minutes of the end of the procedure.
- Advantages:
  - Avoids general anesthesia.
  - Fasting not required.
  - Bloodless operating field.
  - Muscle relaxation.
- Contraindications:
  - Allergy or hypersensitivity to lidocaine.
  - Homozygous sickle cell disease.
  - Severe Raynaud's or Buerger's disease.
  - Crushed or otherwise hypoxic limb.
  - Severe obesity and vascular disease, which a tourniquet could aggravate.
- Risks:
  - Transient paresthesias, mottling, and temperature changes of the limb.
  - Risk of systemic toxicity from premature release of tourniquet.
  - Vasovagal reactions.
- Procedure:
  - Lidocaine *without* epinephrine is the anesthetic of choice. Longer-acting agents such as bupivacaine should *not* be employed.[55]
    - Dilute 1% lidocaine to half strength (0.5% = 5 mg/mL with equal parts of normal saline).
    - Dosage in children and elderly should be 1.5 mg/kg.
    - Dosage in healthy adults can be titrated to 3 mg/kg.
    - In the event that insufficient analgesia is achieved, supplement the intravenous infusion with additional plain normal saline in order to stimulate circulation of the lidocaine within the extremity.
- Equipment:
  - Double-cuff pneumatic tourniquet. *Do not use standard blood pressure cuffs.*
    - The standard blood pressure cuff may suddenly release resulting in a systemic intravascular anesthetic infusion.

- A 50-ml syringe with plastic tube and 22-gauge butterfly needle.
- Cotton or felt cast wrap to pad the limb beneath the tourniquet.
- Cardiac monitoring should be routine.
- Procedure (upper limb):
  - Place the deflated double-cuff tourniquet on the patient's upper arm.
    - ▶ Use cast padding under the cuff to prevent bruising.
  - Insert butterfly cannula (22 gauge or smaller) into a vein on the injured extremity *at least 10 cm distal* to the pneumatic tourniquet and close to the site of injury. Tape in place.
  - Elevate the injured extremity for 3–4 minutes and wrap it from distal to proximal with compression bandage to exsanguinate the limb's blood supply.
  - Inflate the distal tourniquet to about 250–300 mm Hg (patient's systolic blood pressure + 100 mm Hg as guide).
    - ▶ In children, use systolic blood pressure +50 mm Hg.
    - ▶ Avoid this procedure in elderly obese individuals suspected to have significant arteriosclerosis.
  - Infuse the calculated dose of anesthetic via the butterfly catheter.
  - When the infusion is complete, remove the IV cannula and maintain pressure and bandage the IV site.
  - Carry out the procedure.
  - If during the course of the procedure the patient experiences severe pain at the site of the tourniquet, then inflate the proximal tourniquet to the equivalent pressure of the distal tourniquet, and *only* then deflate the distal tourniquet.
  - Once the anesthetic has been infused, the tourniquet *must remain inflated* (either the distal or proximal cuff) *continuously for at least 30 minutes.*
  - Once 30 minutes has elapsed or the procedure has been completed, whichever is longer, *but not more than 60 minutes,* then the tourniquet should be released through a *cycling process:*
    - ▶ Release the pressure on the tourniquet for 5–10 *seconds* and then reinflate the cuff to its occlusion pressure for 1–2 minutes.
      - ○ Repeat this release/reinflate cycle three times in order to prevent a rapid bolus of lidocaine into the systemic circulation.
  - The patient will probably need additional analgesics after the procedure since the lidocaine typically dissipates quickly after tourniquet release.
  - The patient should be observed for at least 30 minutes postprocedure for systemic reactions or toxicity.

Hematoma Block

- Concept: local anesthetic delivered by infiltration directly into the hematoma, which has formed at the site of the fracture.
- Indications:
  - Closed fractures, especially those of the upper extremity.
    - ▶ Do not perform a hematoma block through contaminated or infected soft tissues.

- Advantages:
  - Can be executed very quickly.
  - Avoid procedural sedation.
- Procedure:
  - Prepare the skin site overlying the fracture with antiseptic solution.
  - Inject 5–15 mL of plain 1% lidocaine, or 5–10 mL of plain 2% lidocaine into the hematoma forming at the fracture site and through the disrupted periosteum.
  - In this specific case, aspirate to *ensure* that blood is returned in the syringe, indicating appropriate positioning within the hematoma.
  - Wait 5–10 minutes for onset of block.

Suggested Reading

Amsterdam JT, Kilgore KP. Regional anesthesia of the *head and neck*. In: Roberts JR, Hedges JR, Custalow CB, Chanmugam AS, Chudnofsky CR, McManus LTC, eds. *Clinical procedures in emergency medicine.* Philadelphia, PA: Saunders Elsevier, 2010:500–512.

Barash PG, Cullen BF, Stoelting RK. *Handbook of clinical anesthesia,* 5th ed. Philadelphia, PA: Lippincott Williams & Wilkins, 2006.

Crystal CS, Blankenship RB. Local anesthetics and peripheral nerve blocks in the emergency department. *Emerg Med Clin North Am* 2005;23:477–502.

Crystal CS, McArthur MD, Harrison, B. Anesthetic and procedural sedation techniques for wound management. *Emerg Med Clin N Am* 2007;25:41–71.

Dillon DC, Gibbs MA. Local and regional anesthesia. In: Tintinalli JE, Stapdzynski JS, Ma OJ, Cline DM, Cydulka RK, Meckler GD, eds. *Emergency medicine: a comprehensive study guide.* New York: McGraw-Hill Medical, 2010:270–283.

Farrell RG, Swanson SL, Walter JR. Safe and effective IV regional anesthesia for use in the emergency department. *Ann Emerg Med* 1985;14:239–243.

Karmakar MK, Ho AMH. Acute pain management of patients with multiple fractured ribs. *J Taum* 2003;54:615–625.

Martin B, Ali B. Towards evidence based emergency medicine: best BETs from the Manchester Royal Infirmary. Regional nerve block in fractured neck of femur. *Emerg Med J* 2002;19:144–145.

Melton S, Liu SS. Regional anesthesia techniques for acute pain management. In: Ballantyne JC, Fishman SM, Rathmell JP, eds. *Bonica's management of pain.* Philadelphia, PA: Lippincott Williams & Wilkins, 2009.

Mikrogianakis A, Valani R, Cheng A. *The hospital for sick children manual of pediatric trauma.* Philadelphia, PA:Wolters Kluwer, Lippincott Williams & Wilkins, 2008.

Mohr B. Safety and effectiveness of intravenous regional anesthesia (Bier block) for outpatient management of forearm trauma. *CJEM* 2006;8(4):247–250.

Mulroy MF, Bernards CM, McDonald SB, et al. *A practical approach to regional anesthesia.* Philadelphia, PA: Lippincott Williams & Wilkins, 2009.

Roberts JR, Carney SK. Intravenous regional anesthesia. In: Roberts JR, Hedges JR, Custalow CB, Chanmugam AS, Chudnofsky CR, McManus LTC, eds. *Clinical procedures in emergency medicine.* Philadelphia, PA: Saunders Elsevier, 2010:535–539.

Shanti CM, Carlin AM, Tyburski JG. Incidence of pneumothorax from intercostal nerve block for analgesia in rib fractures. *J Traum* 2001;51:536–539.

Stoelting RK, Miller RD. *Basics of anesthesia,* 5th ed. Philadelphia, PA:Churchill Livingstone Elsevier, 2007.

Wu T, Borock EM. *Digital nerve block.* In: Shah K, Mason C, eds. *Essential emergency procedures.* Philadelphia, PA: Lippincott Williams & Wilkin, 2008.

13 Pediatric Pain Assessment and Nonpharmacological Therapy

Tracy Akitt, Sadie Bartram, Sheryl Christie, and Karen Paling

Introduction

- Many factors can contribute to how a child perceives pain and copes with anxiety-provoking situations.
- The pain response for a particular patient is individual and learned through social learning and experience.
- Unmanaged pain can lead to:
  - Short-term consequences such as children displaying heightened sensitivity to subsequent medical procedures.
  - Long-term consequences such as the development of hyperalgesia.
- Pain endured as a child correlates with adult behaviors such as pain responses, fear, coping effectiveness, and willingness to seek medical attention.

Understanding Coping Mechanisms

- Adequate interventions to assess and manage childhood pain are essential.
- Use a multimodal and multisystem approach when treating a child in pain.
- Involve skilled and specially trained professionals such as child life specialists to assist with pain assessments and interventions, and also to assist pediatric patients and their caregivers to cope.
- Through appropriate assessment, coping behaviors can be identified as to how a child responds to anxiety and distress.
  - According to Kuttner (1996), there are four types of coping behaviors:
    - *Catastrophizers* – view painful events in a very negative way. Although they ask many questions to gain information, the information is not comforting.
    - *Sensitizers* – find the information is comforting to them. They are able to gather lots of information to develop more coping strategies to handle painful events.
    - *Minimizers* – only process information given in small amounts. They are able to use the information to help themselves cope with situations and may require more time to develop coping strategies.
    - *Deniers* – prefer not to have any information. This can be difficult when it is time for the stressful event to occur (i.e., surgery).

- It is important to note that these coping behaviors are not static and can change over time depending on the situation and the supports provided.

Use of Child Life Specialists in the Emergency Department

- Implementing child life programs in the emergency department (ED) have been shown to relieve the stress and anxiety associated with an ED visit.
- Procedure teaching and support, guided imagery, distraction, and other techniques used during procedures have been shown to:
  - Improve coping and decrease upset behavior (of patients and parents).
  - Decrease medication required for sedation or analgesia.
  - Improve staff efficiency.
  - Improve parent satisfaction.

Pediatric Pain Assessment

- Pain assessment in children should be an ongoing process.
- Assessment tools should be used to understand the level of pain a patient is experiencing (see examples listed in Tables 13.1–13.5).
  - Many hospitals have a variety of pain assessment tools readily available for their staff. Check with your local resources.
- Pain in children is measured by:
  - What the child says.
  - What an observer sees.
  - The child's physiological responses to pain.
- A child's cognitive and language development play a large role in their ability to "self-report" pain, thereby making it necessary to rely more heavily on observational and biophysiological measures for infants, toddlers, and patients with neurocognitive impairments.
- Self-reporting considerations:
  - A child's pain is measured simply by asking the child how much he or she hurts, where it hurts, and for how long it has hurt.
  - The child is the best source of information, as he or she is truly the only person who knows the intensity of the pain.
  - A child's self-report, when possible, should be the primary measure of pain assessment.
- Factors that will influence a child's pain response include:
  - Cognitive, emotional, and language development, as this will influence how children perceive and understand pain (see Tables 13.1.–13.5).
  - Developmental age and temperament.
  - Previous pain experiences and a child's memory in relation to these experiences.
  - Caregiver involvement.

TABLE 13.1: Infant pain assessment and nonpharmacological pain management strategies

---

Infant (birth–18 mo)

Cognitive perceptions of pain

0–3 mo
- No apparent understanding of pain; memory for pain likely but not conclusively demonstrated; responses appear mostly reflexive.

3–6 mo
- Response to pain supplemented with sadness and anger.

6–18 mo
- Developing fear of painful situations; early stages of being able to localize pain (through touching/pointing).
- Understanding of common words for pain evolving such as "owie, ouchie, booboo."
- It is important to remember that words for pain vary with cultures and languages.
- Ask parents the words they frequently use at home.

Pain assessment tools

Self-rating – Not possible.
Biophysiological – Heart rate, oxygen saturation, palm sweat.
Observations (behavioral):
- Cry (length and type), facial expressions, body movement, parent ratings/perceptions.
- Neonatal Facial Action Coding System (N-FACS).
- Children's Hospital of Eastern Ontario Pain Scale (CHEOPS) – (1–7 yr).
- Faces, legs, activity, cry, consolability (FLACC) – (0–7 yr).

Considerations for procedural preparation

Information to include:
- Important to prepare the parents of infants. Their comfort to stay during the procedure should be assessed, and their presence should be encouraged.
- Give parents information on the steps of the procedure, the responses their child could exhibit, and where to be positioned during the procedure.

Developmental considerations:
- Infants are at a stage of building a secure attachment to a parent.
- Including parents in all aspects of care and to be their source of comfort is highly important.

Without these interventions:
- Infant's stress levels can increase in absence of nurturing and comforting responses.
- Failing to relieve the pain can cause mistrust and fear toward caregivers.
- Immediate effects such as irritability, fear, and sleep disturbance may occur.
- Effects include delayed healing, impaired emotional bonding, and altered response to subsequent painful experiences.

Environmental considerations

Caregiver involvement:
- Encourage parental participation during the procedure to comfort their child.
- Separation from parents can heighten the distress of infants.
- If the parents are not comfortable or unable to stay, it is important for them to return as quickly as possible.

Health care worker behaviors:
- Changes or missing their usual routine of sleeping, eating, and bathing can be distressing for the child.
- This routine should be respected by the health care workers by planning procedures to be implemented to allow the child's routine to continue as much as possible, and for the child's routine care to be provided by their parents.

Health care setting:
- Keep the room quiet and calm (voices low).
- Minimize the number of people in the room.

(continued)

TABLE 13.1: Infant pain assessment and nonpharmacological pain management strategies (Continued)

Cognitive and behavioral distraction

Comfort suggestions:
- Pacifier, blanket, favorite item
- Swaddling position, massage, touch

Distraction play materials:
- Rattles, pop-up toys, light-up toys, music, bubble blowing

Distraction conversation:
- Singing, action rhymes, positive comforting words

Relaxation methods:
- Massage, touching, blowing bubbles, blowing bubbles away

Developmental Age

- Younger children (younger than 7 years):
  - Rate their pain as higher than older children and display more distress during a painful event.
  - Level of distress and pain ratings may be due to:
    - ▶ Their developmental level of not understanding the purpose of a painful procedure.
    - ▶ The fact that they do not grasp that often the procedural pain will be over quickly.
    - ▶ Their limited ability to use cognitive coping strategies.
- Older children (older than 7 years):
  - Are better able to distinguish the difference between "pain," "unpleasantness," and "fear."
  - May feel a need or may want to appear stoic, thus pain ratings (both self- and observer-reported) may be lower than younger children's pain ratings.

Temperament

- Temperament is a concept defined by Thomas and Chess that describes a person's behavioral style.
- Temperament theory looks at how children will respond to an external stimulus.
  - Three temperament categories are as follows:
    - ▶ Difficult
    - ▶ Easy
    - ▶ Slow to warm up
  - Children considered by parents to have "difficult" temperament were rated as having greater pain responses than children who were found to have "easy" temperaments when requiring immunizations.
- Health care providers need to be flexible and adapt their interventions and modify the environment to better match the child's temperament.

TABLE 13.2: Toddler pain assessment and nonpharmacological pain management strategies

---

Toddler (18 mo–3 yr)

Cognitive perceptions of pain

18–24 mo
- Use the word "hurt" (language/culture specific) to describe pain and noncognitive coping strategies.

24–36 mo
- Beginnings of pain description and attribute an external cause to pain.
- Threat of immediate pain is overwhelming, particularly in situations where the child has a recent previous experience with that same or similar pain stimulus (i.e., IV start or blood work).
- Future benefit of procedure not understood.

Pain assessment tools

Self-rating – Difficult to assess as there is a large developmental range in abilities.
Biophysiological – Heart rate, oxygen saturation.
Observations (behavioral):
- Children's Hospital of Eastern Ontario Pain Scale (CHEOPS) – (1–7 yr).
- Faces, legs, activity, cry, consolability (FLACC) – (0–7 yr).

Considerations for procedural preparation

Information to include:
- Sensations and the steps of the procedure need to be explained to the parents and child.
- Use simple, developmentally appropriate language.
- Allow the child to explore the equipment used for upcoming procedures.

Developmental considerations:
- Toddlers are at a developmental stage where they want to develop a sense of autonomy.
- Allowing toddlers explore the hospital room helps them to express this need for independence.

Without these interventions:
- Can respond with resistance and uncooperativeness.
- Since they can remember painful procedure, they could react the same way in future procedures.

Environmental considerations

Caregiver involvement:
- Allow parents to comfort versus restrain their child during procedures.
- Having comfort items available (e.g., a blanket or stuffed animal) is important when parents cannot be present.
- Allow parents to provide routine (daily) care to their child.

Health care worker behaviors:
- Since toddlers need to feel they are doing things independently, it is important to give the child a role in their health care. It can be something simple like helping put on a blood pressure cuff.
- Minimize the use of restraint. If it is necessary, it should be done seconds before the procedure starts.

Health care setting:
- Exploring the room can be normal behavior for toddlers.
- This curiosity can be used as a means of distraction for the child.
- Keep the room quiet and calm (voices low), and minimize the number of people in the room.

Cognitive and behavioral distraction techniques

Comfort suggestions:
- Pacifier, blanket, favorite item.
- Position of comfort sitting "front to front" or "back to front" in parent's arms, in a chair, or on the bed.
- Massage, touch

Distraction play materials:
- Pop-up books, light-up toys, music, musical/sound toys, motion windup toys

Distraction conversation:
- Singing, action rhymes, storytelling, reading books, counting

Relaxation methods:
- Massage, touching, blowing bubbles, blowing bubbles away

TABLE 13.3: Preschool pain assessment and nonpharmacological pain management strategies

---

Preschool (3–6 yr)

Cognitive perceptions of pain

36–60 mo
- Can give gross indications of the intensity of pain and beginning to use more descriptive adjectives and attach emotional terms such as "sad" or "mad" to the pain.

Pain assessment tools

Self-rating – 36–60 mo – Gross indications of pain (no pain, a little pain, a lot of pain); can mark site of pain on a body outline.
"Poker Chips" – Children (ideally, over 60 mo) are asked to show how much pain they are having by using one to four red poker chips to represent their pain.
"OUCHER" Scale – Used in children over 36 mo in which the children point to one of six faces represented on the scale to indicate which face represents the level of pain they are having.
Biophysiological – Heart rate, oxygen saturation.
Observational (behavioral):
- Children's Hospital of Eastern Ontario Pain Scale (CHEOPS) – (1–7 yr).
- Faces, legs, activity, cry, consolability (FLACC) – (0–7 yr).

Noncommunicating Children's Pain Checklist (NCCPC) – To be used with developmentally delayed children 3–18 yr old.

Considerations for procedural preparation

Providing the information:
- Disseminate the information with the child and parents present.
- Include sensory information and the steps of the procedure.
- Preschool aged children can have the tendency to fantasize information into scary or overwhelming thoughts. Information about procedures should be given immediately before the procedure.
- Be honest with the child about the pain the procedure may cause, but be mindful of the words used.
Special considerations:
- Child may perceive pain as a punishment for something they did wrong. This should be addressed in preparing the child.
- Using real medical equipment in the preparation helps the preschooler to understand and is helpful in detecting the child's fears.
Without these interventions:
- The preschoolers can continue to believe that they have done something wrong, and continue to view the hospital and associated procedures as punishment.

Environmental considerations

Caregiver involvement:
- Allow parents to be the primary source of comfort.
- Parents can also be taught how to encourage the child's coping strategies and utilize distraction techniques (see below) throughout the procedure.
Health care worker behaviors:
- Can engage in simple communications with children of this age. This helps to build rapport and trust with both the child and the parents.
- If restraint is necessary, it is important to tell the child that you are helping them hold still and only do so seconds before the procedure is to start.
Health care setting: Allow the child to explore the room. Keep the room quiet and calm (voices low), and minimize the number of people in the room.

(continued)

TABLE 13.3: (Continued)

Cognitive and behavioral distraction techniques

Comfort suggestions:
- Blanket, favorite item
- Position of comfort sitting "front to front" or "back to front" in parent's arms, in a chair, on the bed, or in sitting position with parent next to child

Distraction play materials:
- Pop-up books, light-up toys, music, musical/sound toys, bubble blowing, motion windup toys, search and find books, videos interactive technology devices

Distraction conversation:
- Singing, action rhymes, storytelling, reading books, counting, talking about favorite things, jokes/humor

Relaxation methods
- Massage, touch, bubble blowing, blowing bubbles away, imagining blowing out candles, imagining blowing up balloon, pinwheel blowing, party blowers
- Guided imagery (imagining a special favorite place)

- It is important to assess and collaborate with parents with regards to how they feel their children's temperament may affect their ability to cope with their pain.

Previous Experience

- The child's previous experience with painful events must be taken into account by health professionals during pain assessment.
- Bijttebier and Vertommen (1998) suggest that a child's pain response is predominantly shaped by the quality of the previous experience than the presence of previous experience with a painful event.
  - History of negative pain experiences:
    - Show higher levels of anxiety before the procedure.
    - Display more distress.
    - Less cooperative during the procedure.
  - History of positive pain experiences:
    - More cooperative.
    - Develop effective coping strategies, which help to reduce pain and allow the child to gain a sense of mastery over the situation.

Memory

- Infants subjected to many painful procedures become conditioned to anticipate pain.
- The memory of a painful event may be distorted, often overestimating the pain felt during the procedure.
- Memories of a painful experience can be reframed, which can help to reduce distress for subsequent procedures.
- Consult a health care professional such as a child life specialist to help the child reframe a painful event, discuss the effectiveness of coping strategies used during the procedure, and set the stage for subsequent procedures.

TABLE 13.4: School age pain assessment and nonpharmacological pain management strategies

---

School age (6–12 yr)

Cognitive perceptions of pain

- Can explain where a pain hurts by grossly explaining and pointing.
- Can explain what happened (history) to better understand what is wrong.

Pain assessment tools

Self-rating – Coping can impact their ability to decipher physical pain and anxiety.
Wong-Baker FACES scale – This scale uses a series of six faces that progressively appear more uncomfortable. The faces also have a numerical value associated with them (0, 2, 4, 6, 8, 10).
"Poker Chips" – See Table 13.3.
"OUCHER" scale – See Table 13.3.
Biophysiological – Heart rate, oxygen saturation.
Observational:
- Children's Hospital of Eastern Ontario Pain Scale (CHEOPS) – (1–7 yr).
- Faces, legs, activity, cry, consolability (FLACC) – (0–7 yr).
- Procedure Behavior Checklist – (6–18 yr).

Noncommunicating Children's Pain Checklist (NCCPC) – To be used with developmentally delayed children 3–18 yr old.

Considerations for procedural preparation

Providing the information:
- Parents should continue to be included in preparation, and involved during the procedure.
- Be open and honest about pain and discomfort that may occur.
- If pain does occur when they have been told it will not, the child may lose trust in the health care worker.
Special considerations:
- At this age, children begin to understand more about pain, but have a fear of death and disability associated with pain.
- Children should therefore be encouraged to ask questions and express feelings.
- Thinking patterns at this age are still very concrete, therefore words should be chosen carefully.
Without these interventions:
- Distress can be indicated by crying, anger, fear, and withdrawal.
- If the child has not been prepared, they may not utilize their coping strategies well and could become more anxious and lose trust in the care providers.
- Explain sensations they will experience during procedures before they occur, allowing time for the child to ask questions.

Environmental considerations

Caregiver involvement:
- It has been thought that children of this age can be without their parents for a longer period of time, but parental presence remains important throughout hospitalization. Because of the psychosocial challenges a hospital visit presents, regression can be seen in the child, and their need for parental presence continues.
- Parents can also play an active role to help their children cope at this age.
Health care worker behaviors:
- This age group is at a developmental stage where they want to develop a sense of accomplishment.
- Should offer choices during the child's hospital stay.
- These choices could include things like choosing to sit up or lay down during a procedure.
Health care setting:
- School-aged children are able to understand the relationship between events and experiences.
- Keep in mind that presenting an IV tray, for example, before being ready to start the procedure could potentially bring about anticipatory anxiety.
- Keep the room quiet and calm (voices low), and minimize the number of people in the room.

(continued)

TABLE 13.4: (Continued)

Cognitive and behavioral distraction techniques

Comfort suggestions:
- Blanket, favorite item
- Position of sitting with parent next to child

Distraction play materials:
- Music, musical/sound toys, bubble blowing, motion windup toys, search and find books, videos, video games, squishy balls, interactive technology devices

Distraction conversation:
- Reality conversation, reading books, counting, talking about favorite things, jokes/humor

Relaxation methods:
- Massage, touch
- Breathing strategies – blowing bubbles, deep breathing, blowing up balloon in stomach
- Guided imagery (imagining a special favorite place)

Caregiver Involvement in Assessment

- When self-report is not possible (child is too young or cognitively impaired), caregivers should be regarded as "the expert" on their child.
- Parents often know their child best and are often able to predict how he or she will respond to pain.
- Parents will also be able to identify some of the words their children use to describe their pain to make a more accurate pain assessment.

Nonpharmacological Pain Management

- It is important to use a combination of nonpharmacological interventions.
- For procedure-related pain in children and adolescents, it is important to use a variety of cognitive behavioral interventions.
- Cognitive behavior strategies:
    - Must be used together, and not in isolation.
    - Can be used for a variety of medical procedures, adapting information appropriately for the different procedures.
- Pain interventions focus on minimizing pain and distress during the procedure by:
    - Creating a positive health care environment.
    - Encouraging parent coaching and involvement.
    - Preparing the child and family.
    - Utilizing cognitive behavioral distraction techniques.
    - Modeling relaxation strategies to aid coping.

Interventions

Health Care/Procedure Environment

- Children may encounter medical procedures for very different circumstances.

TABLE 13.5: Adolescent pain assessment and nonpharmacological pain management strategies

---

Adolescent (12–18 yr)

Cognitive perceptions of pain

■ As children get older, they potentially have more words/experiences to draw upon to better describe the value of their pain (i.e., stabbing/sharp/dull).

Pain assessment tools

Self-rating – Many more self-report tools are available for this age group due to their maturing cognitive abilities. Coping can impact their ability to decipher physical pain and anxiety.
Wong-Baker FACES scale – See Table 13.3.
Biophysiological:
■ Heart rate, oxygen saturation.
Observational:
■ Some adolescents are less likely to verbalize pain, and so lack of crying or moaning in itself should not be used as the only indicator of pain.
■ Procedure Behavior Checklist – (6–18 yr).
Noncommunicating Children's Pain Checklist (NCCPC) – To be used with developmentally delayed children 3–18 yr old.

Considerations for procedural preparation

Providing the information:
■ Parents should be prepared for the responses their child may have to procedures.
■ Increased understanding at this stage, so they may also ask for, and need more details about procedures.
■ Include the steps of the procedure, the sensations to be felt, all while encouraging their questions to be asked.
Special considerations:
■ Adolescents understand more about the emotional and physical aspects of pain and its cause.
■ Have a more sophisticated understanding of the consequences of an injury or procedure and therefore could experience heightened anxiety.
■ Allow time for questions, encourage their participation, and allow some control.
Without these interventions:
■ Because of the loss of independence and control that can result from being in the hospital, adolescents could respond with anger and frustration.

Environmental considerations

Caregiver involvement:
■ Increasing need for a sense of identity and independence can result in ambivalence to their parent's involvement.
■ Adolescents can go from wanting their parents involved to feeling embarrassed about their continued involvement. Wishes for parental or no parental involvement, as well as their privacy, should be respected.
Health care worker behaviors:
■ Health care workers' roles are especially important with adolescents as the establishment of a good relationship facilitates coping and greater cooperation.
Health care setting:
■ Respect privacy, autonomy, and self-respect.

Cognitive and behavioral distraction techniques

Comfort suggestions:
■ Favorite item
■ Provide patient with the choice of parental support
Distraction play materials:
■ Music, search and find books, videos, video games, squishy balls, interactive technology devices
Distraction conversation:
■ Reality conversation, reading books, counting, talking about favorite things, positive self-statements, jokes/humor
Relaxation methods:
■ Massage, touch, progressive muscle relaxation
■ Breathing strategies – deep rhythmic breathing, watching stomach rise and fall
■ Guided imagery (imagining a special favorite place)

- For children experiencing the procedure for the first time, they:
  - ▶ Are often unfamiliar with the setting and will require preparation as to what to expect.
  - ▶ Will benefit from more explanations for various procedures.
  - ▶ Require support for development of new coping strategies.
- Previous experiences or chronic conditions:
  - ▶ Interventions depend on whether the experience was negative or positive.
  - ▶ Often having a familiar health care worker perform the procedure tends to decrease distress.
  - ▶ Require support to accommodate any coping strategies they have used in the past.
  - ▶ Exposure to procedural cues like seeing medical equipment can heighten a child's anxiety; therefore, make accommodations as needed.
  - ▶ Delaying a procedure can also heighten a child's anxiety if they are already prepared and familiar with what is happening.
- Health care workers should take the time to introduce themselves and get to know the child prior to the procedures.
- Keep a calm and quiet environment to alleviate distress.
- Children tend to be less distressed when they have some control over the situation.
  - By giving choices (to watch or look away) and being flexible about utilizing comfort positions such as sitting in a parent's lap or sitting up in a chair can aid in the child being more relaxed and less distressed.
- Children should be allowed to express their pain or discomfort by crying/shouting out as this can also result in less distress during a painful procedure.
- If a procedure is attempted unsuccessfully, then children should be offered the option of taking a break.

Caregiver Coaching/Involvement

- Children perceive parents being present during blood draw to "help the most."
- A parent's comfort level should not be assumed.
  - The parents should always be asked to determine their comfort level to be present during procedures.
  - Parents often feel helpless when observing their child in distress.
  - Parents need to feel empowered and in control of the situation in order to adequately support their child through procedures.
  - It is important to make parents aware that openly displaying emotions reinforces the child's lack of control and emotional reactivity.
- When parents and health care workers are focusing on coping-promoting behaviors, this assures that parents engage in fewer undesirable distress-promoting behaviors and promote more positive outcomes for their child.
  - The distress a child experiences can be affected by any adult responses and comments during a procedure.
  - Parents and health care providers should not focus on the distressing parts of the procedure.
  - Avoid expressing any negative thoughts or feelings about the procedure.

- Parents need preparation and coaching on how to effectively encourage their child's coping strategies.
  - Parents should be given an active role, and be prepared on how they can best help their child.
  - Parent positioning is important to consider.
  - Parents can be educated on the different distraction techniques beneficial for their child's age.
  - Parents can be encouraged to identify that the child is not alone and everyone is working together to minimize the child's pain and anxiety, can aid in calming a child, and reassure them that they are safe and secure (i.e., "we are going to help you get through this").

Positive Reinforcement

- It is important to continue to give praise for positive behaviors before, during, and after the painful procedure.
- It is important to empower the child through positive words and give the child choices so that they can feel they are actively participating in creating a positive outcome.
- Reassurance should be done in combination with other strategies.

Providing Information/Preparation

- Preparation can act as an exposure-based treatment to:
  - Reduce anticipatory anxiety and distress.
  - Reduce fear of the unknown.
- Provide the child and parent with skills to use to cope during the procedure. Children who are well informed about a procedure report less pain than children who do not know the purpose of the procedure.
- Preparations can differ, depending on:
  - Developmental age group.
  - Previous experience.
  - Temperament.
  - Attitude.
  - Coping skills.
- Other factors that are considered when trained professionals, such as child life specialists, are preparing a patient for a procedure include:
  - *Timing of when the information should be provided,* recognizing and allowing time for the children to rehearse and plan coping strategies, and to ask questions.
  - *Language and terminology used,* avoiding medical jargon.
  - *Delivery of information,* presented in a nonthreatening way, the use of sensory information to describe what the child will feel, and the timing and sequence of events.
  - *Tools used,* to include hands-on exploration of equipment kits, and picture preparation books developed for various procedures.
  - *Development of coping strategies,* to include openly talking about feelings, misconceptions, and fears; selection of comfort measures; rehearsal of breathing/relaxation strategies; and selection of distraction techniques.

Behavioral and Cognitive Distraction

■ Cognitive and behavioral distraction involves the use of children's imagination and sense of play.

■ It involves both the use of various play materials (i.e., bubbles, videos, toys) and nonprocedural related conversation (i.e., counting, singing, and discussing favorite things).

■ Used to redirect the child's attention from the painful event.

■ In order for distraction techniques to be effective, these activities must be relevant, developmentally appropriate, and contain observable behaviors.

    ● Giving the child something concrete to focus and specific instructions on what you require them to do is much more effective and will increase understanding and compliance.

Relaxation

Breathing Exercises

■ Promote relaxation.

■ Encourage deep breathing, where the child is moving their diaphragm and exhaling through their mouth, and can elicit more rhythm and pacing for relaxation.

    ● Very young children can also be encouraged to sing, blow bubbles, or pretend to blow out birthday candles as these activities encourage controlled breathing that promotes relaxation and distraction.

Guided Imagery

■ Involves guiding children to use their imagination so that they can focus on feelings that are opposite to the feeling of pain and distress.

■ Guided imagery has been shown to distract and reduce the perception of pain.

Suggested Reading

American Academy of Pediatrics Committee on Psychosocial Aspects of Child and Family Health & American Pain Society Task Force on Pain in Infants, Children, and Adolescents 2001. The assessment and management of acute pain in infants, children, and adolescents. Pediatrics 2001;108(3):793–797.

Bijttebier P, Vertommen H. The impact of previous experience on children's reactions to venepunctures. J Health Psychol 1998;3(1):39–46.

Blount R, Piira T, Cohen L, et al. Pediatric procedural pain. Beh Modif 2006;30(1):24–49.

Carr T, Lemanek K, Armstrong F. Pain and fear ratings: Clinical implications of age and gender differences. J Pain Symptom Manag 1998;15(5):305–313.

Chen E, Zeltzer L, Craske M, et al. Alteration of memory in the reduction of children's distress during repeated aversive medical procedures. J Consul Clinical Psych 1999;67(4):481–490.

Cohen L. Reducing infant immunization distress through distraction. Health Psychol 2002;21(2):207–211.

Cohen L, Blount R, Cohen R, et al. Children's expectations and memories of acute distress: Short- and long-term efficacy of pain management interventions. J Pediatr Psychol 2001;26(6):367–374.

Duff A. Incorporating psychological approaches into routine paediatric venepuncture. Arch Dis Child 2003;88(10):931–937.

Franck L, Greenberg C, Stevens B. Pain assessment in infants and children. Pediatr Clin N Am 2000;47(3):487–512.

Gaynard L, Wolfer J, Goldberger J, et al. Psychosocial care of children in hospitals: a clinical practice manual from the ACCH child life research project. Rockville, MD: Child Life Council, 1998.

Goodenough B, Kampel L, Champion G, et al. An investigation of the placebo effect and age-related factors in the report of needle pain from venipuncture in children. Pain 1997;72(3):383–391.

Goodenough B, Thomas W, Champion G, et al. Unravelling age effects and sex differences in needle pain: ratings of sensory intensity and unpleasantness of venipuncture pain by children and their parents. Pain 1999;80(1–2):179–190.

Kleiber C, Schutte D, McCarthy A, et al. Predictors of topical anesthetic effectiveness in children. J Pain 2007;8(2):168–174.

Kuttner L. A child in pain: how to help, what to do. Vancouver, BC: Hartley & Marks, 1996.

Leahy S, Kennedy R, Hesselgrave J, et al. On the front lines: Lessons learned in implementing multidisciplinary peripheral venous access pain-management programs in pediatric hospitals. Pediatrics 2008;122(3S):S161–S170.

Lee L, White-Traut R. The role of temperament in pediatric pain response. Issues Compr Pediatr Nurs 1996;19(1):49–63.

Mathew P, Mathew J. Assessment and management of pain in infants. Postgrad Med J 2003;79(934):438–443.

Pate J, Blount R, Cohen L, et al. Childhood medical experiences and temperament as predictors of adult functioning in medical situations. Child Health Care 1996;25(4):281–298.

Porter F. Pain assessment in children: infants. In: Schechter NS, Berde C, Yaster M, eds. Pain in infants, children and adolescents. Baltimore, MD: Williams & Wilkins, 1993.

Powers S. Empirically supported treatments in pediatric psychology: procedure-related pain. J Pediatr Psychol 1999;24(2):131–145.

Rollins J, Bolig R, Mahan C. Meeting children's psychosocial needs across the health-care continuum. Austin, TX: Pro-ed, 2005.

Rusy LM, Weisman SJ. Complimentary therapies for acute pediatric pain management. Pediatr Clin North Am 2000;47(3):589–599.

Stanford E, Chambers C, Craig K, et al. "Ow!": spontaneous verbal pain expression among young children during immunization. Clin J Pain 2005;21(6):499–502.

St. Germaine, Brent A. The management of pain in the emergency department. Pediatr Clin North Am 2000;47(3):651–679.

Taddio A, Shah V, Gilbert-MacLeod C, et al. Conditioning and hyperalgesia in newborns exposed to repeated heel lances. JAMA 2002;288(7):857–861.

Young K. Pediatric procedural pain. Ann Emerg Med 2005;45(2):160–171.

Systems Based Approach to Pain Management

14

Headache

David Ng

Epidemiology of Headache

- The prevalence of migraines is 10%–15%, and females are affected three times more than men.
- Patients presenting with headache account for up to 4% of all emergency department (ED) visits.
  - Four percent of headaches have serious or secondary pathology.
  - 0.5% of headaches have life-threatening pathology.
- Twenty-five percent of women and 9% of men experience disabling migraines.
  - Disabling migraines cost 4–6 lost workdays a year, amounting to direct/indirect costs of 17 billion a year in the USA.

Pathophysiology of Headache

- The brain parenchyma is insensate to pain.
- Pain receptors originate in large cranial vessels, venous sinuses, proximal intracranial vessels, pia mater, and dura mater.
- Serotonin (5-HT) receptors are the main focus of pain management as they are known to modulate peptide release and regulate cerebral vessels.
- The anterior vessels are innervated by V1, while the posterior vessels are innervated by C2. Pain can be more generalized or referred to the associated dermatome.
- Pathophysiology of primary headaches remains poorly understood.
  - Current theories of primary headache pathology include:
    - Hypersensitivity of nociception of myofascial tissue.
    - Cortical neuronal depression phenomena.
    - Abnormal vascular dilatation/inflammation.

Classification of Headache

- Classified as either primary or secondary headache as per the International Headache Society (see Table 14.1).
- Primary headache originates from the pain receptors.
  - Although potentially disabling, primary headaches are not life threatening.

TABLE 14.1: Primary and secondary headaches[a]

Secondary headache		Primary headache
Acute danger	Non-acute danger	**Primary headache**
Subarachnoid hemorrhage	Cervical stenosis	Tension
Meningitis	of C2	Migraine
Cerebral venous sinus thrombosis	Trigeminal neuralgia	Cluster
Carotid/vertebral artery dissection	HTN	
Pseudotumor cerebri	Sinusitis	
Glaucoma	TMJ disorder	
Temporal arteritis	Post-lumbar puncture	
Eclampsia	Concussion	
CO poisoning	Medication overuse	
Brain tumor[a]	Brain tumor[a]	
Trauma[a]	Trauma[a]	

[a]Danger is dependent on degree of increased intracranial pressure, shift/effect on intracranial structures due to hemorrhage/mass effect.

- Secondary headache is due to a specific pathology that stimulates the pain receptors.
- It is important to identify which ones are life threatening to the patient.

Goals in the Emergency Department

- Want to rule out all life-threatening secondary causes of headache.
- Key questions to consider on history:
  - Periodicity and how this particular episode evolved.
  - Associated features.
  - Behavior during headache.
  - Family history of migraines and aneurysms.
  - Current medications.
  - Social situation and stressors.
  - What the patient thinks.
- Fundoscopy should be carried out on all patients with headache, along with a neurological exam.
- Patients presenting with the following red flags should have emergency neuroimaging in the ED:
  - New onset headaches.
  - Thunderclap headache.
  - Headache with an atypical aura (lasting over an hour or with motor weakness).
  - Aura without headache in a patient who is migraine naïve.
  - New headache in a patient over the age of 50.
  - Progressively worsening headache.
  - Headaches that change with posture or other maneuvers that increase ICP.

- New headache in a patient with HIV, cancer, or immunodeficiency.
- Headache with fever.
- Headache associated with focal neurological symptoms.
■ Response to therapy should not be an indicator of benign etiology.

Specific Management of Headache in the Emergency Department

Primary Headaches
■ See Chapter 10 on pharmacology of pain management for specific medications.

Tension Type
■ Recurrent episodes that last from hours to days.
■ Typically bilateral, non-pulsating headache with no associated features.
■ Specific treatment:
  - Ibuprofen 200–400 mg, acetaminophen 1 gm q4hr (grade A).
    ▶ NSAIDs (Naproxen 375, diclofenac 25, ibuprofen 400 mg) have similar effect to each other.
  - Caffeine 65 mg PO maybe a useful adjunct, but will increase GI side effects/dizziness (grade B).
  - Ketorolac 60 mg IM for acute relief of moderate to severe headache (grade B).
  - There is no evidence/conflicting evidence for the use of triptans and muscle relaxants.
  - Avoid narcotic, hypnotic combinations due to increased use of overuse, rebound, tolerance/dependency (grade C).

Migraine Type
■ Recurrent attacks that last from 4 hours to 3 days, usually having one to two episodes per month.
  - Patients are asymptomatic between episodes.
■ Typically unilateral, throbbing associated with nausea, vomiting, photophobia (may or may not have aura).
■ Specific treatment:
  - Intravenous fluids and dark/quiet environment.
  - Avoidance of physical activity.
  - If mild, consider NSAIDs, acetaminophen (grade B).
  - If moderate or severe pain, consider triptans or dopamine antagonists, both have about 65–70% response rate (grade A).
  - IV dexamethasone 10–25 mg shows modest effect in decreasing relapse rate at 24–72 hours, NNT = 9 (grade A).
  - If recurrent or disabling, consider prophylactic treatment – beta-blockers, TCAs, SSRIs, anticonvulsants (grade A).
■ Avoid opioids because they have increased risk of rebound headache with return to ED compared to placebo.

Cluster Type

- Short-lasting attacks (anywhere from 15 min to 3 hr), recurring frequently in bouts of 6–12 weeks in a year.
- Typically, severe unilateral orbital, temporal pain lasting 15–180 minutes, associated with ipsilateral lacrimation, rhinorrhea, facial swelling, miosis, and ptosis.
- Specific treatment:
  - High flow O_2 (non-rebreather mask 7–12 L for 20 min) effective in 70% of patients (grade A).
  - Sumatriptan 6 mg SC (grade A).

Specific Anti-migraine Medications

Triptans

- Triptans are serotonin 5-$HT_{1B/1D}$ receptor agonists.
- The choice of Triptan is influenced by onset, route of administration, efficacy, and rate of side effects.
- Triptans are contraindicated in patients with significant coronary artery disease due to vasoconstrictive effects.
- Serious adverse effects include:
  - Coronary artery spasm.
  - Serotonin syndrome.
  - Drug–drug interaction with MAO inhibitors, oral contraceptives, other SSRIs, estrogen-containing contraceptive pills, and CYP3A4 inhibitors.
- Common side effects of triptans include (triptan sensations):
  - Paresthesias.
  - Flushing.
  - Mild neck tightness or chest pressure.
- See Table 14.2.

TABLE 14.2: Pharmacokinetic and efficacy rates of different Triptans

Triptan	Onset	Adverse event rate (%)	Absolute sustained pain-free rate (%)	Special note
Almotriptan 12.5 mg Po	<1 hr	14.2	25.9	Least amount of recurrent headache
Sumatriptan 100 mg po 6 mg sc	1.5 hrs po 15 min sc	33.6	20	Only triptan to have SC and IN routes
Rizatriptan 10 mg	1 hr	40.8	25.3	Comes in oral disintegration tablet
Eletriptan 40 mg	<1.5 hr	42.3	20.9	
Zolmitriptan 2.5 mg	<1.5 hr	39.2	19	IN formulation available

[a]Doses illustrated are maximum single dose, however, a second rescue dose can be administered 2 hours later if headache has not resolved.
SC, subcutaneous; IN, intranasal.

Dopamine Antagonists

■ Choice of medications include (grade A):
  ● Chlorpromazine 10 mg IV.
  ● Metoclopramide 10 mg IV.
  ● Prochlorperazine 10 mg IV.
■ Conflicting studies show chlorpromazine and prochlorperazine to be superior or equivalent to metoclopramide.
■ IM formulation associated with high relapse rate.

Dihydroergotamine

■ Mechanism through alpha receptor blockade and serotonin agonist.
■ Dihydroergotamine (DHE) 1 mg IV q1hr PRN (maximum 3 mg) or 1 spray IN q20min (grade A).
■ Although clinically effective, trials show it to have increased GI side FX and to be inferior compared to dopamine agonists or triptans in efficacy.

Secondary Headaches

■ Need to identify the cause and address with specific treatment.

Subarachnoid Hemorrhage

■ Headache is the predominant symptoms in these patients.
■ Usually a sudden onset headache that reaches peak intensity within a few minutes.
■ Majority of aneurysmal SAH occur between 40 and 60 years with mean age of 50.
■ High mortality up to 50%.
■ Etiology
  ● Eighty-five percent are due to bleeding from a cerebral aneurysm.
  ● Ten percent from non-aneurysmal perimesencephalic hemorrhage.
■ Diagnosis:
  ● Urgent noncontrast CT scan.
    ▶ Sensitivity is up to 98% if performed within the first 12 hours.
  ● If CT scan is negative, then lumbar puncture (LP) is needed to look for red cells and xanthochromia (yellow color caused by breakdown of bilirubin and oxyhemoglobin).
  ● A negative CT and CT-angiogram can exclude subarachnoid hemorrhage with 99% post-test probability.
■ Management:
  ● Neurosurgical intervention of aneurysm.
  ● Management of blood pressure to minimize re-bleeding risk is controversial (given risk of decreased perfusion/increased infarction).
  ● Stop antiplatelet agents and reverse anticoagulation agents.
    ▶ FFP.
    ▶ 10 mg IV vitamin K, prothrombin complex concentrate (octaplex) 40 mL IV.

Thunderclap Headache

- Sudden onset explosive headache.
- Always consider as subarachnoid hemorrhage until proven otherwise.
- Differential diagnosis includes:
  - Cerebrovascular accident.
  - Venous sinus thrombosis.
  - Hypertensive emergency.
  - Cervical artery dissection.
  - Intracranial hypertension.
  - Third ventricle colloid cyst.
  - Intracranial infection.
- Diagnosis:
  - Diagnosis of exclusion.
- Etiology:
  - Probable role of cerebral vasoconstriction and excess sympathetic activity or sensitivity.
- Management:
  - Need to rule out subarachnoid hemorrhage with CT/LP. Consider MRI for venous sinus thrombosis/cervical artery dissection.
  - If workup is negative, and primary thunderclap headache is diagnosed, consider role of sympathomimetics (pheochromocytoma, drug abuse).

Giant Cell Temporal Arteritis

- Usually in patients over the age of 55, mean age of 72 years.
- Incidence of 1/500 for people over 50 years.
- No adverse effect on mortality.
- Fifteen to 20% have permanent vision loss (often at time of presentation)
- Clinical features:
  - New headache over jaw, face, eyes, tongue with features of claudication.
  - Patients may present with systemic symptoms (malaise, polymyalgia, fever).
  - Possible elevated ESR/CRP.
  - Visual changes.
  - Tenderness/decreased pulse over temporal artery.
- Etiology:
  - Chronic vasculitis of medium, large vessels, most commonly cranial arteries originating from aortic arch.
- Diagnosis:
  - Definitive diagnosis is with a positive temporal artery biopsy.
- Treatment:
  - Treat immediately (prior to biopsy) if visual loss or high suspicion.
  - Prednisone 40–60 mg po OD (grade 2c) if no visual loss.
  - Methylprednisolone 1 gm IV (grade 2c) if visual loss.

- ASA 80/100 mg /day (grade 1b).
- Optho/rheum/neuro consultation.

Cerebral Venous Thrombosis

- More common in women (3:1).
- Frequency uncertain, but presumed to be uncommon <1/100,000.
- Estimated 10% mortality if treated.
- Eighty percent have full recovery.
- Pathophysiology:
  - Thrombosis of cerebral veins, dural sinus results in increased venous pressure → cerebral edema/venous hemorrhage → cerebral ischemia
- Risk factors:
  - Prothrombotic conditions (acquired/genetic).
  - Oral contraceptive medications, pregnancy.
  - Malignancy.
  - Infection.
  - Head Injury.
- Clinical presentation:
  - Highly variable.
  - Eighty-five percent of cases present with at least one risk factor.
  - Acute, subacute, or chronic headache.
  - Headache worse with recumbency or Valsalva maneuver.
  - Signs and symptoms of intracranial hypertension, focal neurological deficits, encephalopathy, seizure.
- Diagnosis:
  - MRI is most sensitive.
  - Can use CT with contrast looking at the venous phase.
  - Noncontrast CT – only 70% sensitive.
- Treatment:
  - Anticoagulation with low-molecular-weight heparin/Coumadin.

Post-LP Headache (PLPHA)

- Ten to 30% of patient post-LP will have a headache.
- Pathophysiology:
  - CSF leakage from the dura with traction on pain-sensitive structures.
  - Consider cerebral venous sinus thrombosis (as LP is rare cause of this).
- Clinical features:
  - Typically self-limited.
  - Onset 12–24-hour post-LP, resolves within 14 days.
  - Worse with upright position.
- Prevention/treatment:
  - Use of smaller needle, bevel parallel to longitudinal dura fibers.

- No role for prolonged recumbency in prophylaxis.
- Bed rest and oral analgesics for mild PLPHA.
- Consider caffeine sodium benzoate 500 mg in 1 L NS over 1 hour (grade B).
- Epidural blood patch for severe, refractory PLPHA (grade B).

Trigeminal Neuralgia

- Paroxysms of unilateral facial pain described as an electrical discharge, followed by a brief spasm.
- Follows sensory distribution of trigeminal neuralgia.
- Pathophysiology:
  - Either primary or secondary due to compression from tumor or aneurysm, or chronic inflammation.
- Clinical features:
  - Pain occurs in brief episodes.
  - Usually unilateral.
  - Can have a trigger point along the nerve.
- Prevention/treatment:
  - Carbamazepine 100–200 mg BID (grade A)
  - Other options: Baclofen, Gabapentin, Clonazepam, Amitriptyline.
  - Surgery if nerve decompression is an option.

Medication Overuse Headache

- Occurs when patient takes analgesics frequently for headaches.
- Estimated to happen in 1% of adults.
- Usually occur with overuse of triptans, ergotamines, analgesics, opioids.
- Pathophysiology incompletely understood.
- Diagnosis:
  - Headache presents on ≥15 days/month fulfilling criteria C and D.
  - Regular overuse for ≥3 months of one or more drugs that can be taken for acute and/or symptomatic treatment of headache.
  - Headache has developed or markedly worsened during medication overuse.
  - Headache resolves or reverts to its previous pattern within 2 months after discontinuation of overused medication.
- Treatment:
  - Abrupt withdrawal of analgesia with long-acting NSAID for non-opioid/hypnotic overuse.
  - Consider taper or clonidine and medical observation for high-dose opioid/hypnotic overuse.

Pseudotumor Cerebri (Idiopathic Intracranial Hypertension)

- Annual incidence is 9/1,000,000 in the general population.
  - This increases 20 times in obese women aged 20–44.

- Risk factors:
  - Medications – tetracycline.
  - Female gender.
  - Obesity.
- Clinical features:
  - Papilledema is the hallmark of idiopathic intracranial hypertension (IHI).
  - Chronic headache.
  - Retrobulbar pain.
  - Transient vision loss (75% of patients).
  - Pulsatile tinnitus (60% of patients).
  - Sixth nerve palsy.
- Papilledema can lead to permanent blindness if left untreated.
- Diagnosis:
  - Diagnosis of exclusion: must exclude secondary causes of increased ICP.
  - CT +/− MRI to rule out above.
  - MRI findings include 'empty sella,' dilation of the subarachnoid space around optic nerve, and posterior sclera flattening at the lamina cribrosa.
  - LP with opening pressure >250 mm H_2O.
- Management:
  - Low sodium weight loss program.
  - Acetazolamide 500 mg PO BID.
  - Consideration of: Furosemide 20 mg BID, glucocorticoids, topiramate, TCAs, valproate.
  - Serial LPs for refractory cases.
  - Ophthalmology and neurology referral.

Suggested Reading

Bendtsen L. Central and peripheral sensitization in tension-type headache. Curr Pain Headache Rep 2003;7(6):460–465.

Chronicle E, Mulleners W. Anticonvulsant drugs for migraine prophylaxis. Cochrane Database Syst Rev 2004;(3):CD003226.

Cohen A, Burns B, Goadsby P. High flow oxygen for treatment of cluster headache: a randomized trial. JAMA 2009;302(22):2451–2457.

Colman I, Brown M, Innes G, et al. Parenteral metoclopramide for acute migraine: meta-analysis of randomised controlled trials. BMJ 2004;329(7479): 1369–1373.

Colman I, Brown M, Innes G, et al. Parenteral dihydroergotamine for acute migraine headache: a systematic review of the literature. Ann Emerg Med 2005;45(4):393.

Colman I, Friedman BW, Brown MD, et al. Parenteral dexamethasone for acute severe migraine headache: meta-analysis of randomised controlled trials for preventing recurrence. Br Med J 2008;336:1359.

Goadsby PJ, Lipton RB, Ferrari MD. Migraine: current understanding and treatment. N Engl J Med 2002;346(4):257–270.

Gronseth G; Cruccu G; Alksne J, et al. The diagnostic evaluation and treatment of trigeminal neuralgia (an evidence-based review): report of the Quality Standards Subcommittee of the American Academy of Neurology and the European Federation of Neurological Societies. Neurology 2008;71(15):1183–1190. Epub 2008 Aug 20.

Hu XH, Markson LE, Lipton RB, et al. Burden of migraine in the United States: disability and economic costs. Arch Intern Med 1999;159:813–818.

Jensen R. Peripheral and central mechanisms in tension-type headache: an update. Cephalalgia 2003;23(Suppl 1):49–52.

Kubitzek F, Ziegler G, Gold MS, et al. Low-dose diclofenac potassium in the treatment of episodic tension-type headache. Eur J Pain 2003;7(2):155–162.

Lipton R, Baggish J, Stewart W, et al. Efficacy and safety of acetaminophen in the treatment of migraine: results of a randomized, double-blind, placebo-controlled, population-based study. Arch Intern Med 2000;160(22):3486–3492.

Matthews Y. Drugs used in childhood idiopathic or benign intracranial hypertension. Arch Dis Child Educ Pract Ed 2008; 93(1):19–25.

Miner J, Smith S, Moore J, et al. Sumatriptan for the treatment of undifferentiated primary headache. Am J Emerg Med 2007;25(1):60–64.

Oldman AD, Smith LA, McQuay HJ, et al. Pharmacological treatments for acute migraine: quantitative systematic Review. Pain 2002;97(3):247–257.

Pope JV, Edlow JA. Favorable response to analgesics does not predict a benign etiology of headache. Headache 2008;48(6):944–950.

Prior M, Cooper K, May L, et al. Efficacy and safety of acetaminophen and naproxen in the treatment of tension-type headache. A randomized, double-blind, placebo-controlled trial. Cephalalgia 2002;22(9):740–748.

Ramirez-Lassepas M, Espinosa CE, Cicero JJ, et al. Predictors of intracranial pathologic findings in patients who seek emergency care because of headache. Arch Neurol 1997;54(12):1506–1509.

Tejavanija S, Sithinamsuwan P, Sithinamsuwan N, et al. Comparison of prevalence of post-dural puncture headache between six hour-supine recumbence and early ambulation after lumbar puncture in Thai patients: a randomized controlled study. J Med Assoc Thai 2006;89(6):814–820.

Tomkins G, Jackson J, O'Malley P, et al. Treatment of chronic headache with antidepressants: a meta-analysis. Am J Med 2001;111(1):54–63.

Yucel A, Ozyalcin S, Talu G, et al. Intravenous administration of caffeine sodium benzoate for postdural puncture headache. Reg Anesth Pain Med 1999;24(1): 51–54.

15

Chest Pain

Jessica Hernandez and Jarone Lee

Introduction

- Chest pain accounts for 10% of visits to the emergency department (ED).
- Etiologies of chest pain range from life threatening to benign.
- Forty-five percent of patients with chest pain are eventually diagnosed with acute coronary syndrome.
  - Of these, 7% are younger than the age of 35, and 50% are older than the age of 40.
- Noncardiac causes of chest pain include:
  - GI disease – GERD/reflux, esophageal spasm, peptic ulcer disease, biliary colic, pancreatitis, bowel obstruction.
  - Respiratory – pulmonary embolus, pneumonia, pneumothorax, pleurisy, empyema.
  - Chest wall syndromes – shingles, soft tissue injuries, rib fracture.
  - Nerve root compression.
  - Psychiatric – anxiety, globus, panic disorders, somatization.
- Musculoskeletal pain accounts for 36% of chest pain complaints, of which 13% are due to costochondritis.

Pathophysiology

- Chest pain is frequently described as the following:
  - Tightening, burning, pressure, aching, sharp, tearing, or gaseous.
- Chest pain sensation from visceral organs (esophagus, heart, lung, great vessels, etc.) arise from the same autonomic ganglia.
- Painful stimuli felt in the chest can refer throughout the torso, neck, and upper extremities.
- No one description of chest pain can be definitively correlated with a specific cause.

Cardiovascular Chest Pain
Cardiac Ischemic Pain (Acute Coronary Syndrome)

- Cardiac ischemia is due to an inability to meet oxygen and nutrient demands.
  - Atherosclerosis is the leading cause of coronary vessel narrowing, which leads to ischemia.

- Management:
  - ▶ Percutaneous coronary intervention (PCI) is the management of choice for patients with ST elevation myocardial infarction (MI). In centers without these capabilities, thrombolytics are an option as long as there are no contraindications.
  - ▶ Other management options include:
    - ○ Aspirin – shown to improve mortality with a number needed to treat of 42.
    - ○ Pain control can be achieved with narcotic analgesia and nitrates.
    - ○ Other options have shown no benefit in mortality but are utilized: clopidogrel, glycoprotein IIb/IIIa inhibitors.
- Cocaine-induced chest pain is caused by vasoconstriction of the coronary arteries due to its direct alpha agonist effects. However, it is also known to accelerate atherosclerotic disease.
  - Management:
    - ▶ PCI is the management of choice for patients with signs of ischemia by Electrocardiogram (EKG) and cardiac markers.
    - ▶ Aspirin.
    - ▶ For pain control, consider benzodiazepines, opiates, or nitroglycerin.

Pericardial Pain

- Pericardial pain is caused by inflammation of the pericardial sac (pericarditis).
- Sudden sharp pain that worsens when supine and with inspiration.
- Look for EKG findings or presence of a pericardial rub.
- EKG stages:
  - Stage 1 – diffuse ST elevations with PR segment depression.
  - Stage 2 – normalization of ST and PR changes; flattening of the T waves.
  - Stage 3 – diffuse T wave inversions.
  - Stage 4 – normalization of EKG, or may continue to have persistent T wave inversion.
- Due to its intimate anatomical relationship, myocarditis may also present similarly.
- Etiology includes:
  - Neoplastic.
  - Autoimmune.
  - Infectious – TB, other bacteria, viral.
  - Uremia.
  - Post-MI.
  - Idiopathic.
- Management:
  - NSAIDs are the treatment of choice for these patients.
  - Definitive treatment is varied and should focus on the underlying cause.

Aortic Dissection

- Pain from an aortic dissection occurs when there is a tear in the intimal layer.

- Sudden onset, tearing like sensation.
- Risk factors: elderly patients, hypertension.
- CT angiography is the imaging of choice with high sensitivity and specificity, as well as helping rule out other pathology.
- Classification:
  - Stanford:
    - Type A – involves ascending aorta.
    - Type B – does not involve ascending (arch and descending aorta).
  - DeBakey:
    - Type I – ascending aorta, the arch, and the descending aorta.
    - Type II – ascending aorta only.
    - Type III – distal to left subclavian. Subtype **A** is above the diaphragm and subtype **B** extends below the diaphragm.
  - Management:
    - Management requires tight blood pressure control (Esmolol, Labetalol, or Nitroprusside are the preferred agents).
    - Surgery may be necessary if the tear involves the ascending aorta (Stanford Type A).
    - Manage pain as needed with opiates.

Pulmonary Chest Pain
Pulmonary Embolism

- Pain from pulmonary embolism is caused by the release of inflammatory mediators in the lungs.
- Approximately 10% of pulmonary emboli cause pulmonary infarction, leading to ischemic pain.
- Management:
  - Definitive management is with anticoagulation.
  - Control pain with NSAIDs, acetaminophen, and opiates.

Pneumothorax and Pneumomediastinum

- Pain from spontaneous pneumomediastinum and pneumothorax is due to air leakage into a potential space, which can cause inflammation and compression of surrounding organs.
  - Management:
    - Definitive management may include tube thoracostomy, surgical repair, or observation depending on the size of the pneumothorax and recurrence.
    - Control pain with NSAIDs, acetaminophen, and opiates.

Infectious, Pleurisy, and Pleural Effusion

- Pain due to infections, pleurisy, and effusions is caused by inflammation, and is transmitted via somatic sensation from the parietal pleura.
  - Management:
    - Definitive management may include antibiotics, immunosuppressants, or chemotherapy depending on the underlying cause.
    - Control pain with NSAIDs, acetaminophen, and opiates.

Gastrointestinal Chest Pain
- The most common cause of noncardiac chest pain.

Esophagitis
- The esophagus contains chemoreceptors, mechanoreceptors, and thermoreceptors.
- Esophagitis is caused by inflammation usually due to acid reflux, infection, or ingestion of irritating substances.
  - Management:
    - For infectious esophagitis, pain control is with NSAIDs, acetaminophen, and opiates.
    - Treat underlying etiology with antibiotics, antifungals, or antivirals as appropriate.
    - For gastroesophageal reflux, use acid suppressive therapy such as antacids, H_2 receptor antagonists, and proton pump inhibitors. Also consider prokinetic agents.

Esophageal Rupture
- Esophageal perforation is caused by medical procedures such as endoscopy, over 50% of the time.
- Spontaneous esophageal perforation is commonly due to straining or vomiting, resulting in sudden changes in intraesophageal and intrathoracic pressures causing rupture.
- Leakage of esophageal contents will ultimately cause mediastinal inflammation and pain.
  - Management:
    - Definitive therapy includes broad-spectrum antibiotics and surgical repair.
    - Pain control is with intravenous opiates.

Esophageal Dysmotility (Nutcracker Esophagus, Diffuse Esophageal Spasm, Hypertensive Lower Esophageal Sphincter)
- Esophageal dysmotility disorders cause pain via distention, spasm, or increased intra-esophageal pressures.
  - Management:
    - Calcium Channel Blockers.
    - Other options include:
      - Nitric oxide-based drugs such as nitrates and phosphodiesterase inhibitors.
      - Tricyclic antidepressants.
      - Theophylline.
      - Botox injections.

Musculoskeletal/Neurologic
Trauma, Musculoskeletal, and Costochondritis
- The somatic intercostal nerves perceive muscle exertion, injury to muscle or ribs, and inflammation of the chest wall.

- Management:
  - ▶ Control pain with NSAIDs, acetaminophen, and opiates.
  - ▶ Consider intercostal nerve block (see Chapter 12).

Acute Herpes Neuritis

- Herpes neuritis is an acute reactivation of the varicella virus.
- After reactivation, the virus spreads through the peripheral nerves causing inflammation of skin, soft tissues, and nerves.
- Usually affects one or two adjacent dermatomes on the same side; consider immune-suppressed state if bilateral or multiple dermatomes.
- Most common complication is post-herpetic neuralgia.
  - Management:
    - ▶ If symptoms began within 24–72 hours, consider the use of antivirals.
      - ○ Acyclovir, valacyclovir (pro-drug of acyclovir), or famciclovir can be prescribed for the treatment of herpes neuritis.
      - ○ Brivudine is another antiviral medication available in some countries. Its use is limited due to a potentially fatal interaction with 5-fluorouracil (5-FU).
    - ▶ Control pain with NSAIDs, acetaminophen, and opiates.
    - ▶ For moderate to severe symptoms, consider steroids.

Postherpetic Neuralgia

- Post-herpetic neuralgia occurs when the previously damaged neurons cause spontaneous pain without new injury.
  - Management:
    - ▶ Control pain with NSAIDs, acetaminophen, and opiates.
    - ▶ Typically requires long-term management, with a combination of the following: antidepressants, anticonvulsants, topical capsaicin, MDA receptor antagonists, intrathecal glucocorticoids, cryotherapy, and surgery.

Summary

- Chest pain is a common presentation to the ED with a variety of causes.
- Several life-threatening causes need emergent investigations and specific treatment.

Suggested Reading

Alper BS, Lewis PR. Treatment of postherpetic neuralgia: a systematic review of the literature. J Fam Pract 2002;51(2):121–128.

Castell DO. Diffuse esophageal spasm, nutcracker esophagus, and hypertensive lower esophageal sphincter. In: Basow DS, ed. UpToDate. Waltham, MA: UpToDate, 2010.

Coady MA, Rizzo JA, Elefteriades JA. Pathologic variants of thoracic aortic dissections: penetrating atherosclerotic ulcers and intramural hematomas. Cardiol Clin 1999;17(4):637–657.

Dworkin RH, Johnson RW, Breuer J, et al. Recommendations for the management of herpes zoster. Clin Infect Dis 2007;44(S1):S1–S26.

Imazio M, Demichelis B, Parrini I, et al. Day-hospital treatment of acute pericarditis: a management program for outpatient therapy. J Am Coll Cardiol 2004;43(6): 1042–1046.

James B Wyngaarden, Lloyd H Smith Jr. Cecil textbook of medicine, 22nd ed. Philadelphia, PA: W.B. Saunders, 1985.

Klink MS, Stevens D, Gorenflo DW. Episodes of care for chest pain: a preliminary report from MIRNET. J Fam Pract 1994;38:345.

Mark H. Beers MD, Robert Berkow. The Merck manual, 17th ed. Whitehouse Station, NJ: Merck Research Labs, 1999.

Meisel JL. Diagnostic approach to chest pain in adults. In: Basow DS, ed. UpToDate. Waltham, MA: UpToDate, 2010.

Nelson KA, Park KM, Robinovitz E, et al. High-dose oral dextromethorphan versus placebo in painful diabetic neuropathy and postherpetic neuralgia. Neurology 1997;48(5):1212–1218.

Saadoon AA. Spontaneous pneumomediastinum in children and adolescents. In: Basow DS, ed. UpToDate. Waltham, MA: UpToDate, 2010.

Sengupta JN. An overview of esophageal sensory receptors. Am J Med 2000;108(S4):87S–89S.

Swap CJ, Nagurney JT. Value and limitations of chest pain history in the evaluation of patients with suspected acute coronary syndromes. JAMA 2005;294(20): 2623–2629. Review. Erratum in: JAMA 2006;295(19):2250.

16

Back Pain

Elaine Rabin and Nelson Wong

Introduction

- Acute lower back pain is most commonly defined as lower back pain of less than 6 weeks duration.
  - In the emergency department (ED), patients often present within hours to days of onset of pain.
- Lower back pain has a broad differential diagnosis.
- Eighty-five to 97% of acute low back pain is ultimately determined to be mechanical/musculoskeletal or nonspecific in nature.
  - Treatment goals in these cases include pain relief and restoration of function.

Epidemiology

- Approximately one-fourth of US adults have had an episode of low back pain in the past 3 months.
- It accounts for 3% ED visits/year.
- Burden to society:
  - $84–625 billion annually in direct and indirect costs in the USA.
  - Second most common cause of lost time in the work place affecting 2% of US workforce.
  - Leading cause of work disability in adults less than 45 years.
  - Up to one-third of cases become chronic and last over 1 year, limiting activity in 20%.
  - Five percent of cases account for 75% costs.

Goals in the Emergency Department

- Want to rule out life- and limb-threatening causes of back pain before presuming etiolgy to be musculoskeletal and treating for this.
- Key questions to consider on history:
  - Periodicity and how this particular episode evolved.
  - History of trauma.
  - Associated features – anesthesia, paresthesia, paralysis, fecal incontinence, urinary retention.
  - Associated symptoms – fever, syncope, diaphoresis, nausea/vomiting.

- A complete vascular and neurological examination should be carried out on all patients with back pain.
- Red flags for patients presenting to the ED with back pain:
  - Fever with back pain.
  - Associated neurological symptoms.
  - History of intravenous drug use:
    - History of cancer.
    - Immunocompromised or recent steroid use.
    - Age older than 50 or younger than 17 years.
    - Pain lasting longer than 6 weeks.
- Response to analgesia should not be an indicator of benign etiology.

Pearls

- Routine imaging of uncomplicated lower back pain (i.e., no red flags) is not indicated.
- Many asymptomatic patients will have disc bulges demonstrated on MRI, so disc bulges do not necessarily imply causality, especially without radiculopathy/ sciatica.

Etiology

- Musculoskeletal
  - Muscle spasm/strain
  - Disc herniation with or without sciatic symptoms
  - Spinal stenosis
  - Degenerative joint disease
- Urologic
  - Renal colic (see Chapter 21)
  - Pyelonephritis
- Vascular
  - Aortic dissection
  - Epidural hematoma
  - Abdominal aortic aneurysm
- Infectious
  - Spinal epidural abscess
  - Osteomyelitis

Workup for suspected life- and limb-threatening etiologies of Back Pain in the Emergency Department

Cauda Equina Syndrome

- Symptoms due to compression of lower spinal nerve roots.
- Can result from compression for any reason (tumor, hematoma, etc.), but is often due to large intervertebral disc bulge into the spinal canal.

- Signs/symptoms:
  - New, progressive or severe lower extremity motor or sensory deficits.
  - Saddle anesthesia.
  - Urinary retention or incontinence.
  - Decreased rectal tone, bowel incontinence.
- Investigations:
  - If suspected, MRI without contrast is the preferred imaging technique.
  - CT without contrast may be useful if MRI is unavailable.

Abdominal Aortic Aneurysm Rupture

- Risk factors:
  - Older age.
  - Male.
  - Hypertension.
  - Smoking.
  - Atherosclerotic disease.
- Signs/symptoms:
  - Aneurysm without rupture is often asymptomatic.
  - Sudden-onset, colicky pain not related to movement.
  - Hematuria.
  - Classic triad of hypotension, abdominal or back pain, and pulsatile abdominal mass is found in less than half the cases.
  - Common clinical scenario is an older patient presenting with symptoms of renal colic without a previous history of nephrolithiasis.
  - Investigations:
    - ▶ Ultrasound is useful for detecting aneurysm and large amounts of fluid due to rupture.
    - ▶ CT scan with intravenous contrast can reveal both aneurysms and rupture.

Malignancy, Primary Tumor or Metastases

- Primary tumors of the spine are most often lymphoma, leukemia, myeloma, ependymomas and other gliomas.
- Metastases are often due to prostate, breast, and lung cancers.
- Risk factors: Older age, cancer history.
- Signs/symptoms:
  - New back pain in patients younger than 18 or older than 50.
  - Worse lying or sitting, and straining.
  - Gradual onset, unrelieved with medications.
  - Pain at night.
  - Radicular or cauda equina symptoms.
  - Systemic signs of malignancy (e.g., unexplained weight loss, fever).
- Investigations:
  - If suspected, MRI with and without contrast is preferred.
  - CT can be useful if MRI unavailable.

Fractures
- Due to osteoporosis, trauma, or tumor (pathological).
- Risk factors:
  - Cancer.
  - Osteoporosis.
  - Age greater than 50.
  - Recent trauma.
  - Prolonged steroid use.
- Signs/Symptoms:
  - Midline tenderness.
  - Radicular symptoms (particularly in compression fractures due to osteoporosis).
  - Neurologic deficits corresponding to a lesion at a particular spinal level.
- Investigations:
  - X-ray is usually sufficient for diagnosis.
  - Refer for further imaging if pain persists.
  - MRI without contrast is preferred to CT if available.

Abscess (Epidural or Paraspinal)
- Risk factors:
  - Intravenous drug use.
  - Diabetes.
  - Immunocompromised state.
  - Recent epidural anesthesia/injection.
  - Recent proximal skin abscesses
- Signs/symptoms:
  - Fever.
  - Leukocytosis.
  - Radicular or cauda equina symptoms.
  - Paralysis (late-stage finding).
- Investigations:
  - If suspected, obtain MRI with and without contrast if available.
  - Otherwise CT with and without contrast for immediate diagnosis.

Management of Acute Musculoskeletal Lower Back Pain
- Important facts regarding the available evidence:
  - Few rigorous studies on treatment are available.
  - Available studies are mostly from primary care and other office-based literature.
  - Even those focusing on acute lower back pain often study time frames for pain relief not useful for ED visits (days to weeks).
- In practice:
  - 80% of patients are prescribed medications, and more than one-third of patients are prescribed more than one medication.
  - Education is a fundamental part of treatment.

Treatments That Have Been Demonstrated to be Effective

■ Acetaminophen
  ● Few strong studies available.
  ● Compared with NSAIDs:
    ▶ Mixed evidence regarding relative effect (weaker analgesic effect according to data extrapolated from osteoarthritis studies
    ▶ Safer side-effect profile in most patients.
  ● Given favorable side-effect profile and low cost may be considered first-line treatment.
■ NSAIDs
  ● Best-studied class of medications.
  ● Strong evidence of small improvements in the short term.
  ● Onset within 1–2 hours.
  ● No differences found among NSAIDS in effectiveness.
  ● Compared to opioids:
    ▶ Overall evidence is that NSAIDs may be equally effective and generally have a more favorable side-effect profile.
    ▶ In one of the few ED-based studies, ketorolac and acetaminophen-codeine had similar effects, but ketorolac had fewer adverse effects.
  ● Side effects:
    ▶ The lowest effective dose should be used to minimize side effects.
    ▶ Gastrointestinal (GI), renal, and cardiovascular.
      ○ GI side effects are minimal at nonprescription doses.
      ○ Other side effects include abdominal pain, diarrhea, edema, dry mouth, rash, dizziness, headache, and tiredness.
  ● Evidence supports effectiveness in chronic pain as well.
  ● Not helpful if sciatic symptoms are present.
■ COX-2 Inhibitors
  ● COX-2 inhibitors may have equivalent efficacy and fewer GI side effects than other NSAIDs, but have not been well studied to date.
  ● May have increase cardiovascular disease risk.
■ Muscle relaxants
  ● This category is based on the FDA-approved indication; mechanism of action varies and includes centrally acting antispasmodics and peripherally acting antispasticity agents.
  ● Antispasmodics
    ▶ Strong evidence of clinical improvement, especially in the short term for patients without sciatica.
    ▶ Cyclobenzaprine and tizanidine are the most well-studied.
    ▶ No difference has been found among antispasmodic agents.
  ● Less evidence is available for antispasticity agents.
  ● Compared with NSAIDs: may be more effective but the evidence is still unclear.
  ● Combined with NSAIDs:

- ▶ Unclear whether more effective than NSAIDs alone.
- ▶ Combination is associated with an increased frequency of side effects.
- Not a first-line agent for acute low back pain, most often considered an adjunct to analgesics.
- Side effects:
  - ▶ CNS: sedation, dizziness, headache, blurred vision.
  - ▶ GI: nausea and vomiting.
  - ▶ Use of some may lead to dependence.
  - ▶ Various drug-specific serious side effects.
- Benzodiazepines
  - No FDA approval for lower back pain.
  - Compared with muscle relaxants: small number of studies report similar or less effectiveness to skeletal muscle relaxants, however, not all studies demonstrated benefit.
  - Given risks of dependence and inadequate evidence for chronic lower back pain it is not recommended for long-term use.
  - Side effects:
    - ▶ Sedation.
    - ▶ Respiratory suppression.
- Opioids
  - Few trials and no systematic reviews.
  - No differences found among specific opioids.
  - Generally considered effective.
  - Due to side effects and potential for abuse, most guidelines and systematic reviews recommend as second line and for limited course of treatment for acute lower back pain refractory to previous therapy.
  - Compared with NSAIDs: mixed evidence regarding whether more effective (see above).
  - Side effects:
    - ▶ GI: nausea, vomiting.
    - ▶ Sedation and respiratory suppression.
    - ▶ Potential for abuse in patients predisposed to addiction.
    - ▶ Potential for dependence.
- Tramadol
  - Centrally acting with some effect at mu receptors.
  - Similar to opioids: effective for pain relief but with less GI effect and dependence.
  - Side effects: headache, nausea.
- Superficial heat (heating pad, heat wrap)
  - Heat wrap significantly reduced pain versus placebo.
  - Some evidence that 8-hour heat wrap may be more beneficial than NSAIDS, acetaminophen.
  - No risk of systemic side effects.

■ Rapid return to normal activity within the limits of pain.
  ● Universally recommended in published guidelines.
  ● Evidence supports improvement in pain relief and functional status.

Treatments That Have Been Demonstrated to be Ineffective
■ Exercise
■ Bed rest
■ Systemic corticosteroids

Treatments with Unclear Effectiveness
■ Systemic and local steroid injection.
  ● Use reserved for the treatment of epidural compression syndromes with consultation.
■ Transcutaneous electrical nerve stimulation (TENS).
  ● Local electrodes placed overlying skin that deliver electrical stimulation.
  ● Widespread use as a treatment modality for over 30 years.
■ Topical NSAIDs.
■ Topical anesthetics.
  ● Lidocaine patches caused dizziness in some patients.
■ Cold treatment.

Disc Herniation and Spinal Stenosis
■ For disc herniation: look for radicular symptoms, positive straight leg raise.
■ Not as much evidence available regarding therapy, but most symptoms resolve with similar treatment to above in 4 weeks.
■ NSAIDs not better than placebo in patients with sciatica.
■ Acute pain of spinal stenosis may be relieved with walking or exercise.
■ If patient presents with at least 1 month duration of pain, and if the patient is a candidate for epidural injections, discectomy (disc herniation), or spinal surgery (spinal stenosis), consider referral for nonemergent MRI.

Chronic Lower Back Pain
■ Acute on chronic exacerbations of low back pain often present to the emergency room.
■ Studies of low back pain agree that chronic low back pain often tends to be multifactorial in nature.
■ Antidepressant drug therapy has been shown to be useful in some patients, specifically those with underlying depression. The evidence is mixed with regards to patients without underlying depression.
■ Short-term therapy with opioids has been recommended in various clinical practice guidelines.

Suggested Reading

Arnou J, et al. A critical review of guidelines for low back pain treatment. Eur Spine J 2006;15(5):543–553.

Chou R, Huffman LH. Medications for acute and chronic low back pain: a review of the evidence for an American Pain Society/American College of Physicians clinical practice guideline. Ann Intern Med 2007;147(7):505–514.

Chou R, et al. Diagnosis and treatment of low back pain: a joint clinical practice guideline from the American College of Physicians and the American Pain Society. Ann Intern Med 2007;147(7):478–491.

Clark E, Plint AC, Corell R, et al. A randomized, controlled trial of acetaminophen, ibuprofen and codeine for acute pain relief in children with musculoskeletal trauma. Pediatrics 2007;119(3):460–467.

Dagenais DC, Tricco A, Haldeman S. Synthesis of Recommendations for the assessment and management of low back pain from recent clinical practice guidelines. Spine J 2010;10(6):514–529.

Dagenais S, Caro J, Haldeman S. A systematic review of low back pain cost of illness studies in the United States and Internationally. Spine J 2008;8(1):8–20.

Dahm KT, Brurberg KG, Jantvedt G, et al. Advice to rest in bed versus advice to stay active for acute low-back pain and sciatica. Cochrane Database Syst Rev 2010;(6):CD007612.

Davies RA, Maher CG, Hancock MJ. A systematic review of paracetamol for non-specific low back pain. Eur Spine J 2008;17(11):1423–1430.

Deshpande A, Furlan A, Mailis-Gagnon A, et al. Cochrane Database Syst Rev 2007;(3):CD004959.

Deyo RA, Weinstein JN. Low back pain. N Engl J Med 2001;334(5):363–370.

Deyo RA, Mirza SK, Martin B. Back Pain prevalence and visit rates: estimates from us national surveys. Spine 2006;31(23):2724–2727.

French SD, Walker CM. Reggars JW, et al. Superficial heat or cold for low back pain. Cochrane Database Syst Rev 2006;(1):CD004750.

Innes GD, Croskerry P, Worthington J, et al. Ketorolac versus acetaminophen-codeine in the emergency department treatment of low back pain. J Emerg Med 1998;16(4):549–556.

Khadilkar A, Odebiyi DO, Brosseau L, et al. Transcutaneous electrical nerve stimulation (TENS) versus placebo for chronic low-back pain. Cochrane Database Syst Rev 2008;(4):CD003008.

Machado LA, Camper SJ, Herbert RD, et al. Analgesic effects of treatments for non-specific low back pain: a meta-analysis of placebo-controlled randomized trials. Rheumatology 2009;48(5):520–527.

McCarberg BH. Acute back pain: benefits and risks of current treatments. Curr Med Res Opin 2010;26(1):179–190.

Pitts SR, Niska RW, Xu J, et al. National hospital ambulatory medical care survey: 2006 emergency department summary. Natl Health Stat Report 2008;7:1–38.

Reishaus E, Waldbaur H, Seeling W. Spinal epidural abscess: a meta-analysis of 915 patients. Neurosurgical Rev 2000;23(4):175.

Roelofs PD, Deyo RA, Koes BW, et al. Non-steroidal anti-inflammatory drugs for low back pain. Cochrane Database Syst Rev 2008;(1):CD00396.

Stewart W, Ricci J, Chee E, et al. Lost productive time and cost due to common pain conditions in the us workforce. JAMA 2003;290(18):2443–2454.

Van Tulder MW, Touray T, Furlan AD, et al. Muscle relaxants for non-specific low-back pain. Cochrane Database Syst Rev 2003;(2):CD004252.

17

Sickle Cell Pain

Jeffrey Glassberg and Patricia Shi

Epidemiology

- Sickle cell disease (SCD) affects nearly 100,000 individuals in the United States.
- The most common reason for emergency department (ED) visits in this population is vaso-occlusive crisis (VOC).
  - Second most common reason for ED visits is fever.
- In both the ED and inpatient setting, pain is often undertreated.

Pathophysiology

- A point mutation at codon 6 of the β-globin gene causes production of abnormal hemoglobin called hemoglobin-S.
- When both inherited β-globin genes carry this mutation, or the hemoglobin S mutation is paired with another mutation (hemoglobin C and β-thalassemia are the most common), the patient will have SCD.
- In response to tissue hypoxia and stress response, HbS forms rigid polymers, which give erythrocytes their sickle shape.
- The pathophysiology of SCD and its complications are due to many factors including:
  - Enhanced leukocyte activation
  - Increased platelet activation
  - Blood cell adhesion
  - Endothelial dysfunction
  - Chronic hemolysis
- The clinical manifestations are myriad and include:
  - VOC
  - Acute chest syndrome (ACS)
  - Splenic or hepatic sequestration
  - Stroke
  - Aplastic crises
  - Dactylitis
  - Priapism
  - Leg ulcers
  - Increased infection risk – rule out sepsis with fever

- Avascular necrosis
- Bony infarcts and osteomyelitis
- Retinopathy
- Pulmonary hypertension
- The most common manifestation is pain (VOC).
- Most patients experience daily pain, with the most common sites being the lower back and legs.
  - Pain can also progress to VOC where the severity of pain requires high-dose opiates, usually necessitating hospital admission.

Potentially Life-Threatening Causes

- In a patient presenting with pain, all the non-SCD-related, life-threatening causes of pain in that region must be considered (e.g., right lower quadrant pain in a patient with SCD is still appendicitis until proven otherwise).

Acute Chest Syndrome

- It is a serious pulmonary complication, and should be considered in any sickle cell patient presenting with chest pain.
- Overall incidence of 10.5 per 100 patient years.
- Most common in the 2–4 years age group.
- ACS is defined as new infiltrate on chest x-ray with one of the following:
  - Chest pain
  - Fever
  - Respiratory symptoms – dyspnea, tachypnea
  - Hypoxia
- While ACS criteria are not distinguishable from the definition of pneumonia, it is described as a specific entity because:
  - The cause of ACS is not always infection.
  - Etiology is multifactorial:
    - Microbial infection
    - Vaso-occlusion
    - Fat embolism from ischemic/necrotic bone marrow
    - Thromboembolism
  - The treatment for ACS is transfusion or exchange transfusion. Without this, clinical status often deteriorates rapidly with very high mortality.
- Pearl: ACS is usually not the presenting complaint. More commonly, it develops during the course of in-patient admission. Assess frequently for signs and symptoms of ACS.
- Management:
  - Supportive measures – oxygen.
  - Appropriate hydration – avoid bolus of fluids. Consider maintenance fluids without risking overhydration.
  - Appropriate pain control.

- Incentive spirometry.
- Antibiotics: third-generation cephalosporin, macrolides.
- Simple or exchange transfusion.

Vaso-occlusive Crisis
- Hallmark clinical manifestation of SCD.
- Caused by local ischemia from:
  - Decreased blood flow
    - Polymerization of HbS
    - Cellular dehydration
    - Increased vascular adhesion
  - Inflammation
- Precipitants include:
  - Infection
  - Fever
  - Acidosis
  - Hypoxia
  - Dehydration
  - Sleep apnea
  - Extremes of heat and cold
  - Asthma exacerbation
- Clinical presentation:
  - Tenderness
  - Swelling
  - Warmth
- Need to distinguish it from osteomyelitis and septic arthritis. This can be difficult with routine blood work or x-rays. Best option is arthrocentesis for differentiating from septic arthritis and MRI for osteomyelitis.
- It is the most common reason for hospital admission in sickle cell patients.
- Effective management must include:
  - Assessment of pain
  - Treatment of the pain appropriately
  - Frequent reassessment
  - Adjustment of pain medications as necessary
- Barriers to pain management:
  - Limited knowledge of SCD
  - Inadequate assessment of pain
  - Biases against opioid use, with unsubstantiated fear of:
    - Tolerance
    - Dependence
    - Addiction
    - Drug seeking

- Assessment
  - Identify pain location(s)
  - Determine severity
    - Use a validated pain assessment tool. The most common is the 11-point numerical rating scale (0–10), although many others exist.
  - Analgesics used prior to arrival
    - It is crucial to ask the type and dose of analgesics used prior to arrival in order to calculate an appropriate analgesic starting dose in the ED.
  - Potential triggers:
    - See list above.
  - Laboratory evaluation:
    - VOC may be associated with significant changes in hemoglobin levels, hemolysis, and reticulocytosis.
    - Table 17.1 provides a summary of appropriate lab testing during VOC.
  - Pearl: Obstructive lung disease patterns and airway hyperresponsiveness are very common in children with SCD.
    - This is a frequent trigger for VOC.
    - Assess vigilantly for wheezing even if the patient does not carry a diagnosis of asthma and have a low threshold for treating with steroids and bronchodilators.
    - Pain may be more difficult to control if asthma exacerbation is present and not treated.
- Treatment (see Table 17.1)
  - IV fluids:
    - Always use hypotonic IV fluids (e.g., D5½ NS), unless the patient is overtly hypovolemic (e.g., diarrhea).
    - Avoid overhydration as this can potentiate atelectasis, which is associated with the development of ACS.

TABLE 17.1: Management of acute pain crisis

- Labs:
  - CBC, reticulocyte count
  - ALT, LDH, fractionated bilirubin if worsened icterus
  - Type & screen if Hb $\geq$1 g/dL is below baseline
- D5½ NS with 20 mEq KCl/L at 1–1½ times maintenance (100–150 mL/hr)
  - Reassess every 24 hr
- Quickly achieve and maintain pain control
- Adjuvant analgesics: acetaminophen and diphenhydramine/hydroxyzine
- Laxatives: docusate and senna
- Deep venous thrombosis prophylaxis with low-molecular-weight or regular heparin
- Pulse oximetry only to keep O_2 saturation $\geq$92%
- Incentive spirometry with chest or back pain
- Continue outpatient folate and hydroxyurea

- IV opiates
  - ▶ Intravenous opiates (morphine, hydromorphone, and fentanyl) are the cornerstone of pain management for VOC.
  - ▶ At some centers, hydromorphone is preferred due to its low side-effect profile and lack of active metabolites. Selection of opioid is institution and physician dependent.
  - ▶ Meperidine is not recommended and, in patients with renal insufficiency, it is contraindicated due to its active metabolite normeperidine, which causes seizures.
  - ▶ Initial IV opiate dosing should be adjusted based on outpatient usage.
  - ▶ In the initial phase, reassess pain every 15–30 minutes and redose opiates until pain is controlled.
  - ▶ Pain usually improves after two to three doses of IV opiates if administered in rapid succession.
  - ▶ After relief is obtained, it must be maintained with round-the-clock opiate dosing, not just on a prn basis. Two options are listed in Table 17.2, along with tapering recommendations.
  - ▶ Pearl: Do not start PCA until the patient's pain has been controlled by an initial bolus (or boluses) of IV opiates.
    - ○ Without this, the PCA will be inadequate.
    - ○ Weaning should occur after the first 24 hours and be started in the mornings rather than evenings.
  - ▶ Adjuvant medications
    - ○ Acetaminophen and diphenhydramine are indicated because they have opiate sparing effects.
    - ○ Long-term NSAID use should be avoided.
      - ➢ Single bolus dose ketorolac has shown some potential. Further studies are needed in its use.
      - ➢ NSAID use may hasten decline in renal function, especially if renal dysfunction is already present.
      - ➢ Creatinine is not a reliable indicator of subtle renal dysfunction in patients with SCD. SCD patients have supranormal proximal tubule function, which can result in normal creatinine values even when significant renal dysfunction is present.

TABLE 17.2: Around the clock options for adults (>50 kg)

Patient controlled analgesia (PCA) with hydromorphone (1 mg/mL)	Basal 0.1 mg/hr Demand 0.1–0.3 mg q8 min
Long-acting opioid agonist (controlled-release morphine or oxycodone or transdermal fentanyl)	Base initial dosing on short-acting opioid requirements. Rescue doses of 10–15% of the total 24-hr dose or 50% of the 4-hr dose should be the same opioid as the ATC medication, available q1–2 hr prn
Tapering opioids	Wean dose by 10–20% every 8 hr as tolerated to keep pain score <5. Once opioid dose 25–30% of initial level, can switch to equianalgesic oral opioids and consider discharge

▶ Incentive spirometry is indicated for all patients with VOC.
▶ DVT prophylaxis: heparin or low-molecular-weight heparin.
  ○ Low-molecular-weight heparin has been shown to safely reduce the severity and duration of painful crises.
  ○ Unless contraindicated, it should be administered to all admitted patients.
▶ Supplemental O_2 only to keep oxygen saturation above 92%.
▶ Transition to oral opiates.
  ○ When PCA dosing is at 25–30% of its initial level, the patient can be transitioned to oral opiates.
  ○ If the patient prefers a longer acting opiate, start it several days before discharge because it may take three to four doses to reach steady state levels.

Priapism

■ Mean age of onset is 12 years.
■ Occurs as a result of VOC of the penis, which causes obstruction of the venous drainage.
■ Classification:
  ● Prolonged if it lasts more than 3 hours
  ● Stuttering if it lasts for a few minutes, lasts less than 3 hours, and resolves spontaneously
■ Complications of recurrent episodes include fibrosis and impotence.
■ Identify the following at time of presentation:
  ● Time of onset
  ● Last episode and treatment
  ● Trauma
  ● Infection
  ● Drug use – sympathomimetics, alcohol, phosphodiesterase inhibitors
■ Treatment:
  ● Fluids – if prolonged, then consider IV fluids
  ● Analgesia – consider parenteral analgesia (see Section on Vaso-occlusive crisis and Chapter 10)
  ● Alpha agonists (pseudoephedrine 30–60 mg PO)
  ● Beta agonists (Terbutaline 5–10 mg PO)
  ● Aspiration of corpus cavernosum

Suggested Reading

Bellet PS, Kalinyak KA, Shukla R, et al. Incentive spirometry to prevent acute pulmonary complications in sickle cell diseases. N Engl J Med 1995;333:699–703.

Glassberg J, Spivey JF, Strunk R, et al. Painful episodes in children with sickle cell disease and asthma are temporally associated with respiratory symptoms. J Pediatr Hematol Oncol 2006;28:481–485.

Hassell KL. Population estimates of sickle cell disease in the U.S. Am J Prev Med 2010;38:S512–S521.

McClish DK, Smith WR, Dahman BA, et al. Pain site frequency and location in sickle cell disease: the PiSCES project. Pain 2009;145:246–251.

National Institutes of Health. The Management of sickle cell disease, 4th ed. Bethesda, MD: National Heart, Lung, and Blood Institute, 2002:59–74. NIH Publication 02-2117.

Qari MH, Aljaouni SK, Alardawi MS, et al. Reduction of painful vaso-occlusive crisis of sickle cell anaemia by tinzaparin in a double-blind randomized trial. Thromb Haemost 2007;98:392–396.

Smith WR, Penberthy LT, Bovbjerg VE, et al. Daily assessment of pain in adults with sickle cell disease. Ann Intern Med 2008;148:94–101.

Tanabe P, Myers R, Zosel F, et al. Emergency department management of acute pain episodes in sickle cell disease. Acad Emerg Med 2007;14:419–425.

18 Dental and Ocular Pain

Tomislav Jelic, Hareishun Shanmuganathan,
Christian La Rivière, and Shelly Zubert

Dental Pain

Epidemiology

- Dental complaints represent 0.4–10.5% of emergency department (ED) visits.
- Dental complaints can be categorized as (1) orofacial pain, (2) orofacial trauma, and (3) infections.
- Traumatic causes are often secondary to falls, accidents, assaults, or motor vehicle collisions.

Orofacial Pain

- Dental caries
- Periodontal disease (gingivitis)
- Postextraction alveolar osteitis (periosteitis/dry socket)
- Postoperative pain
- Acute necrotizing ulcerative gingivitis (Vincent disease)
- TMJ dysfunction

Orofacial Trauma

- Dentoalveolar trauma
- Dental fractures
- Concussions/luxations/avulsions
- Facial fractures
- Soft-tissue lacerations
- TMJ dislocation

Infections

- Dental abscesses
- Ludwig angina
- Deep neck abscesses
- Cellulitis

Clinical Assessment of Dental Pain

- Before instituting analgesia in any form ensure that cause of pain has not compromised airway:
  - Sublingual hematoma
  - Expanding hematoma
  - Brawny neck (Ludwig angina)
  - Trismus
  - Drooling
  - Neck immobility

Dental Caries

- Represents the loss of integrity of the tooth enamel.
- Pain management consists of oral NSAIDs.
- Regional block may be appropriate in select situations.
- Management consists of ruling out other causes (i.e., abscess) and referral to a dentist.

Postextraction Alveolar Osteitis

- Otherwise known as dry socket, caused by disruption of the clot from the socket, exposing alveolar bone.
- Presents in 2–5% of extractions, usually 3–4 days afterwards.
- Pain management consists of NSAIDs, regional nerve block, and oil of cloves.
- Regional nerve blocks are often required to provide normal saline irrigation and application of packing.
- Antibiotics may be required and referral to a dentist within the next 24 hours.

Dental Abscess

- Secondary to bacterial infection (*Streptococcus* species and oral anaerobes) from untreated dental caries.
- Left untreated can spread to deep neck spaces.
- Regional nerve blocks for the affected region are appropriate within the ED.
- NSAIDs with the possibility of an opioid are also appropriate in pain control management.
- Definitive management includes incision and drainage, tooth extraction, and antibiotics.

Ludwig's Angina

- Infection of submental, sublingual, and submandibular spaces, with elevation and displacement of the tongue, which can lead to airway compromise.
- Poor dental hygiene, dysphagia, odynophagia, trismus, and edema are common signs and symptoms.
- Pain management consists of opioids with close monitoring of airway compromise.
- Regional blocks are not indicated in this condition.
- Definitive management includes IV antibiotics, and emergent referral to ENT for surgical intervention as indicated.

Acute Necrotizing Ulcerative Gingivitis

- Also known as Trench mouth.
- Triad of pain, ulcerated interdental papillae, and gingival bleeding.
- Etiology is poorly understood, but associated in immunocompromised hosts, with *Treponema, Fusobacterium, Selenomonas,* and *Prevotella* commonly found.
- Pain management consists of systemic opioids, oral rinses with viscous lidocaine.
- Definitive management includes warm saline rinses, chlorhexidine rinses, and appropriate antibiotics.

TMJ Dislocation

- Secondary to direct trauma, laxity of ligaments of joint, extreme opening of the mouth, dystonic reactions.
- Anterior dislocation of the condyles that become trapped in the anterosuperior eminence.
- Previous dislocations predispose to further episodes.
- Definitive management of joint reduction will provide analgesia.
- Proper reduction will often require procedural sedation to alleviate pain, muscle spasm, and patient resistance.

Mandibular/Maxillary Fractures

- Pain management consists of systemic opioids and the use of regional nerve blocks where indicated.
- Management consists of ensuring there is no airway compromise and prompt referral to a maxillofacial surgeon.

Tooth Avulsions, Concussions, and Luxations

- Secondary to falls, direct trauma, sporting injuries.
- Definitions:
  - Concussion – no displacement or loosening of teeth. There is crush injury to adjoining tissue.
  - Luxation – dislocation of teeth.
    - ▶ Can be intrusive, extrusive, lateral, lingual, or buccal.
  - Avulsion – loss off tooth from the socket.
- Regional nerve block in the ED may provide the most comfort for the patient (see Chapter 12).
- NSAIDs, soft diets are appropriate as outpatient pain management.
- Stabilization of the tooth and referral to a dentist is required.

Dental Fractures

- Secondary to falls, direct trauma, and sporting injuries.
- Seventy percent is to the central incisors.
- Ellis classification:
  - Class I – involves only the enamel
  - Class II – exposure of the dentin
  - Class III – fracture that includes exposure of the pulp
  - Class IV – root fracture

- Regional nerve block in the ED may provide the most comfort for the patient.
- NSAIDs, soft diets are appropriated as outpatient pain management.
- Referral to a dentist is required for both cosmetic and structural repairs.
- Higher Ellis class requires more urgent referral.

Considerations for Anesthesia for Dental Pain

- Does the patient have any allergies?
- Are they on anticoagulation?
- Is there a need for immediate homeostasis?
- How long is analgesia required?
- What are the requirements for postprocedural analgesia?

Analgesia Options for Dental Pain

- Procedural sedation.
  - Consider use in TMJ dislocation.
- Topical anesthesia.
  - Available in many preparations (e.g., liquids, sprays, and viscous gels).
- Gels are shown to be more effective in providing pain control.
  - Benzocaine (6–20%).
- Rapid onset: ~30 seconds.
- Duration: 5–15 minutes.
- Poor systemic absorption.
  - Lidocaine (2–5%)
- Onset: ~2–5 minutes.
- Duration: 15–45 minutes.
  - Injectable anesthetics
- Determine if large area is required (i.e., nerve block vs. local infiltration) – see Chapter 12 for nerve blocks.
- Recommend topical anesthetic to be applied to area of injection to decrease pain of injection.

Specific Dental Blocks

- See Chapter 12.
- Supraperiosteal Injection.
  - Indication:
    - Provides anesthesia to one tooth (pulp, root, buccal mucosa) for fractures, subluxations, and dry sockets.
- Greater palatine nerve block.
  - Indication:
    - Palatal laceration, maxillary teeth anesthesia.
    - Affects posterior aspect of unilateral hard palate and overlying soft tissues.

- Nasopalatine block.
  - Indication:
    - Augmentation of supraperiosteal injection of the anterior maxillary teeth, and anesthetize anterior palatal mucosa for palatal laceration repair.
    - This block will affect the anterior portion of the hard palate, from the left to right premolars.
- Infraorbital nerve block.
  - Indication:
    - Useful for repairs of area from lower eyelid, lateral nose, and upper lip, as well as providing anesthesia to incisors and canines.
    - Provides anesthesia to the anterior superior, middle superior alveolar nerve, and the infraorbital nerve.
- Inferior alveolar nerve block.
  - Indication:
    - Useful for dry socket pain, postextraction pain, or pulpitis.
    - Anesthesia to unilateral aspect of mandible, mandibular teeth, anterior two-thirds of the tongue and floor of the mouth.
- Supraorbital nerve block.
  - Indication:
    - Forehead and upper eyelid repair.

Ocular Pain

Epidemiology
- Two percent of ED patient visits are for various ocular complaints including primary ophthalmologic, infectious, and traumatic causes.
- Primary complaints include:
  - Glaucoma.
  - Infectious causes include conjunctivitis, herpetic infection, stye, chalazion, periorbital/orbital cellulitis, and corneal ulcer.
  - Traumatic causes include subconjunctival hemorrhage, corneal abrasion, and foreign body.

Considerations in the Management of Ocular Pain
- History or contact with herpes
- Chemical exposure
- Contact lens use
- Ruling out foreign body
- Treating underlying condition (glaucoma)
- Providing systemic/topical antibiotics
- Providing tetanus immunization for abrasions

Clinical Assessment of Ocular Pain

- Before instituting analgesia in any form ensure that vision-threatening diagnosis is ruled out:
  - Retinal artery or vein occlusion
  - Open/closed angle glaucoma
  - Temporal arteritis
- Ensure that complete ophthalmic examination is preformed. This may include:
  - Visual acuity
  - Intraocular pressure
  - Funduscopy
  - Visual fields
  - Pupils
  - Extraocular movements
  - pH
  - Slit lamp with fluorescence

Glaucoma

- Increased intraocular pressure as a result of either overproduction or decreased resorption of aqueous humor.
- As pressure increases, irreparable optic nerve damage can occur.
- Use of NSAIDs and/or opioids systemically in conjunction with treatment to decrease intra-ocular pressure (IOP).
- Management of increased IOP:
  - Carbonic anhydrase inhibitors (Acetazolamide) – decrease aqueous production.
  - Topical beta-blockers (Timolol) – decrease aqueous production.
  - Hyperosmotic agents (Glycerin, Mannitol) – causes fluid shift from eye space into the vascular space, resulting in an osmotic dieresis.
  - Miotic agents (pilocarpine) – causes ciliary muscles to contract thus opening the space in the trabecular meshwork to allow increased absorption of aqueous humor.

Conjunctivitis

- Caused by either bacterial (*Streptococcus pneumoniae, Haemophilus influenzae, Neisseria gonorrhoeae*) or viral infection.
- For pain management, use topical NSAIDs, such as 0.5% ketorolac.
- Anti-histamines can be used for pruritus, which is common in viral conjunctivitis.
- Treat respective infections with appropriate antibiotics.

Herpes Zoster Ophthalmicus

- Rash that follows dermatomal lines.
  - Look for Hutchinson's sign with lesions at the tip of the nose.
- Dendritic like lesions are seen using fluorescein staining.
- Regional blocks can provide temporary relief.

- If pain is ongoing, opioids, tricyclic antidepressants, or gabapentin can be used to decrease duration or severity of post-herpetic neuralgia.
- Requires urgent ophthalmologic consultation requiring intravenous antivirals.

Stye/Chalazion/Blepharitis

- Common presentation to urgent care clinics.
- Generally, secondary to staphylococcal infection.
- Warm compress to affected eye helps alleviate symptoms.
- Treatment with antibiotic ointments and "no tears" shampoo.

Corneal Abrasion

- Defect of the normal corneal epithelium caused by trauma (fingernail, twig, etc. or after foreign body removal).
- Account for up to 10% of eye complaints.
- Topical anesthetics are helpful for pain control in the ED.
- The use of antibiotic ointments and anti-inflammatory eye drops (ketorolac 0.5%, diclofenac 0.3%) are helpful for pain management as well as for the treatment of the underlying condition.
- Eye patches are not indicated. A meta-analysis demonstrated no difference in healing and no reduction in pain.

Corneal Ulcer

- Corneal infection often secondary to contact lens use.
- Pseudomonas very common in this type of infection.
- Topical anesthetics may be used initially in the ED but should not be continued. They are likely to make the ulcer worse.
- Fluoroquinolone eye drops are required q1h. Cycloplegic drops may also be used for pain management.
- Eye patching should not be used!
  - Patching does not reduce pain in adults or pediatric population, and may exacerbate the underlying condition (corneal abrasion, ulcers).
  - There is little role for eye patching in the ED.
- Referral to an ophthalmologist on an emergent basis.

Foreign Body

- Need to rule out possibility of globe injury (e.g., high-velocity metal piece).
- Topical anesthetic very helpful in the ED.
- Must ensure removal of foreign body by examining entire eye including under the lids.
- Irrigation initially may be helpful. Often using a small gauge needle or a burr is required.
- As for corneal abrasions, antibiotic and anti-inflammatory ointments may be helpful.

Topical Agents for Ocular Pain

Artificial Tears

- Two drops 4–6×/day as needed.
- Duration of use should be limited.

Topical NSAIDs

■ Useful in inflammatory changes such as conjunctivitis.

■ Avoid in corneal ulcerations and herpetic infections.
  ● Diclofenac at 0.1% (1–2 drops TID-QID)
  ● Ketorolac 0.5% (1–2 drops TID-QID)

Topical Glucocorticoids

■ Useful in acute anterior uveitis, conjunctivitis, episcleritis, and scleritis.

■ Should only be employed after other treatments have been exhausted.

■ Prolonged use associated with increased risk of cataracts, glaucoma, and infection.
  ● Fluorometholone 0.1% (1 drop BID-TID)
  ● Prednisolone 1.0% (2 drops QID)

Topical Cycloplegics

■ Useful in conditions where blepharospasm is present.

■ One percent cyclopentolate.

Topical Anesthetics

■ Useful in acute ED setting.

■ Should not be prescribed as outpatient as it carries a high risk of secondary keratitis.

Summary

■ Review anesthetic considerations for each patient, to help guide what type of anesthetic/analgesic would be most beneficial for your patient.

■ Consider nerve blocks, as they require less anesthetic, less distortion to tissues, and provide good anesthesia if done correctly.

■ Do not forget to treat the underlying cause of pain.

■ IV opiates should be used in certain cases where other means of analgesia will not be sufficient enough.

■ Topical anesthetics for ocular pain are useful in the acute setting, but patients should not be discharged with them as they carry a high risk of complications with prolonged use.

Suggested Reading

Alteveer J, McCans K. The red eye, the swollen eye, and acute vision loss: handing non-traumatic eye disorders in the ED. Emerg Med Pract 2002;4(6):1–26.

Benko K. Acute dental emergencies in emergency medicine. Emerge Med Pract. 2003;5(5):1–19.

Benko K. Fixing faces painlessly: facial anesthesia in emergency medicine. Emerg Med Pract 2009;11(12):1–19.

Marx JA, Hockberger RS, Walls RM. Rosen's emergency medicine, 7th ed. Philadelphia, PA: Mosby Elsevier, 2009.

19   Prehospital Pain Management

Michelle Welsford and Greg Soto

Introduction

- When it comes to managing acute pain emergency prehospital practitioners, similar to emergency department (ED) personnel, are often falling short.
- Inadequate analgesia, referred to as oligoanalgesia, remains a major problem in both prehospital and Emergency Department (ED) care.
- Inadequate pain control takes several forms:
  - Delayed or nonreceipt of analgesia
  - Use of ineffective analgesia (e.g., non-steroidal anti-inflammatory drugs (NSAIDs) where opioids are indicated)
  - Underdosing analgesics
  - Failure to combine analgesics
  - Failure to use adjuncts
- Two important reasons not to delay analgesia in the field are as follow:
  - Analgesia administration is associated with decreased need for subsequent opioids.
  - If analgesia is delayed until ED arrival, time to administration can be significantly delayed (up to 2 hours in one study).
- Pain is associated with increased morbidity:
  - Increased patient suffering from the unpleasant experience.
  - Can lead to delayed wound healing.
  - Increased metabolic rate.
  - Altered immune response.
  - Lowered pain threshold for subsequent painful experiences.
  - Increased association with PTSD.
- The goal of prehospital pain management is to start the pain relief (not necessarily eliminate) – without significant complications.
- Several important emergency medical service (EMS) advocacy groups have called for improvements in prehospital pain management.
  - The National Association of EMS Physicians, the American College of Emergency Physicians, and the EMS Outcomes Project have all advocated for this.

Reasons for Oligoanalgesia

- Reasons cited for inadequate pain management in the out-of-hospital setting include:
  - Poor understanding of pain
  - Underestimation of pain
  - Poor assessment (poor understanding of available pain assessment tools)
  - Provider biases – barriers such as sex, age, race, ethnicity, language, and socioeconomic status
  - Fears related to opioid dependence and drug-seeking behavior
  - Poor choice of analgesic
  - Inadequate protocols
  - Online medical control physician attitudes and practices
    - ▶ Concern of on scene delay

Pain Assessment Tools

- Patients may not receive analgesia if they are not questioned regarding their pain.
- Emergency providers often underestimate a patient's analgesic requirements.
  - Have also been found to discredit patients' pain based on their own beliefs.
- Pain should be assessed and reassessed to ensure appropriate treatment.
- There are multitudes of pain scales tested and used in hospitals but pain scales used prehospital need to be simple, quick, and reliable.
- The verbal rating scale (VRS) and numerical rating scale (NRS) have both been validated in the ED for adults and have been shown to be easy, quick, discriminating, and reliable.
  - The NRS is likely the most commonly used tool for pain assessment and reporting in prehospital care because it does not require any equipment or charts.
  - Provider verbally asks the patient to rate their pain on a scale of 0–10.
- For children, there are several scales including the pictorial Faces Pain Scale, and for younger children observational/behavioral scales can be used (see Chapters 13 and 22).

Patient Monitoring for Analgesia Administration

- In addition to assessing the patient's perception of pain, it is important for prehospital providers to undertake a full assessment.
  - This includes:
    - ▶ Vital signs prior to analgesia administration (blood pressure, heart rate, respiratory rate, SpO_2, and ECG rhythm).
    - ▶ Continually reassess the patient's pain scores.
    - ▶ Repeat vital signs periodically following analgesia administration.
- It has been established that prehospital providers do not consistently document pain encountered in the field.

- It is important to document:
  - Initial pain score – identifies need for analgesia.
  - Response to initial treatment.
  - Ongoing need for further treatment.
- Knowledge of the side effects of the specific agents will also guide the reassessments so that these can be recognized early and managed (e.g., respiratory depression, hypotension, or nausea and vomiting with opioids).

Contraindications and Cautions for Analgesia Administration

- There are several relative contraindications to administration of analgesics in the field:
  - Hypotension
  - Hemodynamic instability
  - Allergies
  - Comorbidities that can lead to complications with specific agents (e.g., renal failure and NSAIDs)
- Extra caution with above contraindications is necessary in the prehospital setting since there is:
  - Less availability of backup
  - Fewer reversal agents available
  - Fewer agents to counteract complications
- There are also some medical conditions that are best treated with other therapies rather than only analgesics.
  - For example, ongoing cardiac ischemia where treating with analgesics alone may prevent administration of other more suitable medications.

Quality Improvement and Medical Oversight in Pain Management

- Quality improvement programs have been shown to improve assessment of pain and better medical directive compliance.
- Quality improvement programs should include initial and ongoing education and retrospective review to assess if management is appropriate and effective.
- Education should involve:
  - The role of prehospital pain management
  - The assessment of pain severity
  - Nonpharmacologic approaches to pain management
  - Pharmacology of analgesics
  - Patient monitoring and assessment
  - Management of side effects or complications

Nonpharmacologic Pain Management

- There are several nonpharmacologic adjuncts that EMS providers can utilize to reduce pain.

- Therapeutic communication techniques can be used very successfully to calm, provide reassurance, and/or distract the patient.
  - ▶ This may involve reassurance, guided imagery, or breathing techniques.
  - ▶ These techniques are rarely formally taught at present, but rather are part of the "art" of paramedicine and commonly used by experienced EMS providers.
- Distraction such as music can also be used successfully for procedures that are mildly/moderately painful such as IV initiation or wound cleansing/dressing.
- Physical modalities such as splinting/immobilization and/or positioning/ elevation of an extremity may reduce the pain associated with an injury.
- Heat or cold application can modulate pain perception in many injuries.
  - ▶ Heat application has also been shown to dramatically reduce pain in prehospital patients with presumed biliary colic.
- Rubbing, massaging, or providing stimulation to an area proximal to the injury may sometimes reduce the perception of pain in the cerebral cortex (updated gate theory).

Pharmacologic Pain Management
- See Chapter 10.

Opioids
- Commonly used for moderate to severe pain.
- Usually administered intravenously in the prehospital care system with relatively quick onset and ability to titrate to effect.
- Morphine and fentanyl are the most common prehospital opioids.
- Since there are no significant differences in outcomes with morphine and fentanyl, most prehospital systems should choose only one agent, however, the few differences between them may be used to determine preference in specific situations.
- Naloxone is an opioid reversal agent that has significant prehospital experience showing that it is safe and can reverse the respiratory depression and apnea side effects.
- Widespread abuse of opioid medications means that the security of these medications and the safety of the providers is an additional concern.
- Federal legislation governs the storage and procurement of these medications making them more administratively complex.

Morphine
- Most commonly used opioid in prehospital care.
- May also be administered intramuscularly and subcutaneously, but this results in a delayed onset, less agility with titration, and a prolonged action.
- In addition to its use for painful injuries or other truncal pain, it is also commonly used for cardiac ischemic pain when nitroglycerin is not effective.

Fentanyl
- Although fentanyl is less commonly used by ground ambulances, it is as effective as morphine and may have a few advantages.

- Fentanyl is not commonly used for cardiac ischemic pain that is nonresponsive to nitroglycerin not because of concern of poor outcomes, but rather lack of evidence of benefit.
- Shorter duration of action compared to morphine makes it more preferential for procedural or short-term pain and/or for patients whose hemodynamic status may change (severe trauma patients).
- Additional route of intranasal administration makes this agent potentially attractive for pediatric use (no need for intravenous initiation).

NSAIDs and ASA

- These agents are infrequently used by EMSs.
  - Oral preparation results in delayed onset.
  - Usually for mild to moderate pain only.
- Single dose or acute use for most patients is very safe with GI upset and nausea being the most common side effects and renal failure/dysfunction being rare with single acute use.
- NSAIDs are contraindicated in patients with allergies (caution due to ASA and NSAID cross-reactivity allergies including those patients with asthma and atopy).
- There are no reversal agents for NSAIDs.
- There are many concerns with chronic use or in some patients with comorbidities such as risk of GI bleed, renal dysfunction, and potential cardiovascular risks.
- ASA is commonly used by prehospital providers for its anti-platelet actions for patients with possible acute coronary syndromes but not as an analgesic.
- There are no specific monitoring requirements for NSAIDs other that usual reassessment of the patient and their pain.

Acetaminophen

- Similar to NSAIDs, acetaminophen is available in oral forms only in North America.
- Is commonly used for mild to moderate pain although it can be combined with opioids such as codeine, oxycodone, or tramadol to be used for moderate to severe pain.
- Its oral formulation and onset of action limits its use and practicality in prehospital care.

Nitrous Oxide

- Nitrous oxide is an inhaled agent administered as a 50/50 nitrous oxide/oxygen mixture that has analgesic, sedative, and dissociative actions.
- Time of onset is 3–5 minutes with duration of action of 3–5 minutes.
- It requires a tank and special mask with demand valve that allows the patient to self-administer. Patients should receive supplemental oxygen as well.
- The mask must not be secured to the face, but rather self-administered by the patient.
  - As the patient experiences adequate analgesia and/or sedation, the mask will fall from the patient's face preventing oversedation.

- Nitrous oxide is commonly used by EMS services, but there are some concerns that have led to its removal by some EMS providers and/or entire states/provinces.
  - Concern of exposure to ambient gas in the closed space of an ambulance (chronic exposure has been linked to health effects), and the abuse potential by providers.

Pharmacologic Adjuncts to Pain Management

- Sedative agents such as benzodiazepines (lorazepam, midazolam, diazepam) may be used in conjunction with other analgesics by prehospital providers for some emergency procedures (cardioversion, pacing, etc.).
  - It is important to know that these agents are *not* analgesics and should be used with analgesics for painful procedures.
- Other adjunctive medications include some antinauseants used with opioids, where the analgesic effect is additive.
- The effects on sedation, respiratory depression, and blood pressure are additive with opioids and so must be used cautiously.

Prehospital Sedation

- Indications for sedation:
  - Procedural sedation: cardioversion, transcutaneous pacing, intubation (pre and/or post).
  - Pain management adjunct: splinting, extrication, etc.
  - Management of pharmacologic toxicity and/or withdrawal: sympathomimetic toxicity, depressant/alcohol withdrawal.
  - Anxiolysis.
  - Pharmacologic restraint in combative and psychotic patients.
- Contraindication and cautions for sedation:
  - Prehospital sedation uses similar medications as in the ED, but the environment is vastly different.
  - As opposed to the ED, prehospital sedation is usually accomplished by only one (or occasionally two) provider that is responsible for the medication, monitoring, and procedure.
  - The prehospital environment has the additional restrictions of the following:
    - Limited space
    - Limited backup medications
    - Limited backup equipment
    - Lack of backup personnel
  - Therefore, prehospital sedation should be done very cautiously and only when necessary for life-threatening conditions (cardioversion of an unstable rhythm) or for the provider's safety (combative patient).
  - Only providers with education and experience in advanced airway management and ventilation should administer sedation.

- Prehospital drug-assisted intubation (DAI) requires special caution.
  - ▶ The National Association of EMS Physicians Position Statement on the topic recommends that DAI can be harmful and should not be for all providers, but rather only for specially trained and supervised providers that have additional education and CQI.
- Patient care monitoring should include everything discussed under the analgesia section including continuous ECG rhythm, oxygen saturation, HR, RR, and BP, and may also include end-tidal CO_2.

Nonpharmacologic Approach to Anxiolysis

- There are therapeutic techniques, which will assist and enhance sedation although these focus more on reassurance, calming, and guided imagery.
- In the prehospital setting these may not be effective alone for procedural sedation, but they may be invaluable in the anxious patient.

Pharmacologic Agents for Sedation

- See Chapter 3.

Benzodiazepines

- Central neuronal inhibition causing sedation, anxiolysis, and anticonvulsant activity.
- Dosage is very individual and must be titrated carefully to effect.
- Larger doses can cause respiratory depression or excessive sedation requiring intubation although the dosages where this occurs have a wide variation.
- Midazolam may be the ideal agent for prehospital use because of its short onset, short duration, and multiple routes for administration.
- Routes include IV, IO, IM, intranasal, and buccal (between the teeth and the cheek).
- Other agents include lorazepam and diazepam.

Opioids

- As discussed earlier, these agents are analgesics but can also provide some sedation.

Nitrous Oxide

- As discussed above, this agent is useful as an analgesic and also has sedative and dissociative properties but with very short duration of action, so only useful for very short procedures (splinting).

Ketamine

- Little EMS use/experience except in physician-based EMS systems.
- Has analgesic properties at lower doses and dissociative properties at higher doses; does not inhibit respiratory drive and protective reflexes.
- Also has a mild bronchodilatory action, which has lead to its use for intubation induction in asthmatic patients in hospital.
- Can be administered IM and IV.

Suggested Reading

Alonso-Serra HM, Wesley K. NAEMSP position paper: Prehospital pain management. Prehosp Emerg Care 2003;7(4):482–488.

Bredmose PP, Lockey DJ, Grier G, et al. Pre-hospital use of ketamine for analgesia and procedural sedation. Emerg Med J 2009;26(1):62–64.

Fleischman RJ, Frazer DG, Daya M, et al. Effectiveness and safety of fentanyl compared with morphine for out-of-hospital analgesia. Prehosp Emerg Care 2010;14:167–175.

Hennes H, Kim MK. Prehospital pain management: current trends and future direction. Clin Pediatr Emerg Med 2006;7:25–30.

Holbrook TL, Galarneau MR, Dye JK, et al. Morphine use after combat injury in Iraq and post-traumatic stress disorder. New Engl J Med 2010;362:110–117.

Jennings PA, Cameron P, Bernard S. Measuring acute pain in the prehospital setting. Emerg Med J 2009;26(8):552–555.

Kober A, Scheck T, Tschabitscher F, et al. The influence of local active warming on pain relief of patients with cholelithiasis during rescue transport. Anesth Analg 2003;96(5):1447–1452.

Lord B, Cui J, Kelly AM. The impact of patient sex on paramedic management in the prehospital setting. Am J Emerg Med 2009;27:525–529.

McEachin CC, McDermott JT, Swor R. Few emergency medical services patients with lower-extremity fractures receive prehospital analgesia. Prehosp Emerg Care 2002;6:406–410.

McManus JG, Sallee DR. Pain management in the prehospital environment. Emerg Med Clin N Am 2005;23:435–431.

Ricard-Hibon A, Chollet C, Belpomme V, et al. Epidemiology of adverse effects of prehospital sedation and analgesia. Am J Emerg Med 2003;21(6):461–466.

Thomas SH, Shewakramani S. Prehospital trauma analgesia. J Emerg Med 2008;35(1):47–57.

Turturro MA. Pain, priorities and prehospital care. Prehosp Emerg Care 2002;6:486–488.

Wang HE, Davis DP, O'Connor RE, et al. Drug-assisted intubation in the prehospital setting (resource document to NAEMSP position statement). Prehosp Emerg Care 2006;10(2):261–271.

Trauma and Musculoskeletal Pain

Tomislav Jelic, Hareishun Shanmuganathan,
Christian La Rivière, and *Shelly Zubert*

General Principles in the Trauma Patient

- Trauma management should include appropriate pain management for the patient.
- See Chapter 8 on the neurobiology of pain and its effects.
- Effects of uncontrolled pain include:
  - Stress response – sympathetic and catabolic drive.
    - Tachycardia.
    - Increased tissue oxygen consumption.
    - Hypercoagulability.
    - Immunosuppression.
    - Activation of inflammatory mediators.
    - Hyperglycemia.
  - Increased thromboembolic events.
  - Agitation.
  - Pulmonary complications (acute lung injury, acute respiratory distress syndrome).
  - Infections.
  - Increased length of stay.
  - Increased mortality.
  - Increased risk of chronic pain syndromes and posttraumatic stress disorder.
  - Difficulty in managing physiological parameters of the patient, including:
    - Ventilator intolerance.
    - Hemodynamic instability.
    - Gastrointestinal dysfunction.
    - Renal dysfunction.

Stable Trauma Patient

- The first priority is to ensure that the airway, breathing, and circulation are adequate.
- By definition, a stable patient has vitals that are stable and are close to/at the normal limits, GCS 13–15.
- No acute organ dysfunction.

Nonpharmacological Measures

- Patient reassurance.
- Patient positioning.
  - Keep weight off of the injured area.
  - Protect the injured area.
    - ▶ For example, dressings or clean drapes over wounds.
- Supporting the injured area.
  - Splints/supportive bandages or tapes.
  - Backslabs or casts.
  - Elevating injured extremities (when possible) to decrease edema.
- RICE (rest, ice, compression, elevation).

Pharmacological Pain Management

- Assess the patient for allergies or potential drug interactions.
- Use the WHO Analgesic Ladder.
  - For mild to moderate pain, you can start with PO medications first, beginning with acetaminophen or NSAIDs.
  - If pain is severe, use IV medications, titrated to effect to achieve analgesia with minimal side effects (remember that there is no hard-and-fast dose "ceiling" with opioids).
- To maintain analgesia, ensure that the patient is on regular pain medication, and avoid playing "catch up."
- Frequent reassessment of pain and overall clinical status is the key.
- Specific recommendations:
  - IV boluses, repeated every 5–15 minutes, of morphine, fentanyl, and hydromorphone to achieve rapid pain control (see Chapter 10 on pharmacology of pain management).
  - Maintain ongoing analgesia with regularly scheduled doses of IV or PO morphine or hydromorphone.
    - ▶ Fentanyl, while having less cardiorespiratory effects than morphine, is typically too short acting to achieve ongoing pain control, unless an IV infusion is started.
    - ▶ Consider the use of patient-controlled anesthesia (PCA) (see Chapter 10 for PCA choices).
- See Chapter 10 on the side effects of narcotics.
- Trauma pearls:
  - Do not use transdermal opioids (i.e., the fentanyl patch) as absorption of the drug in the acute trauma patient will vary considerably.
  - Do not use extended-/sustained-release opioid drugs in the acute setting as analgesia requirements will vary considerably in the acute setting and the risk of opioid overdose is significant.
  - The application of regional blocks for specific injuries will often reduce the amount of systemic analgesia that is required (see Chapter 12 for specific regional nerve blocks).

Unstable Trauma Patient

- As earlier, securing and maintaining the ABCs take priority over analgesia.
- By definition, an unstable trauma patient has disrupted vitals, severe ongoing hemorrhage, and/or evidence of acute organ dysfunction.
- Nonpharmacological measures as described above are the first step.
- Consider regional blocks as they avoid the side effects of systemic opioids (pruritus, hypotension, respiratory depression), however, they introduce the risks of local anesthetic toxicity and peripheral nerve injury.
- Need to balance pain control with ongoing management and side effects of the medications.
- Parenteral therapy is preferred for moderate to severe pain.

Ketorolac

- Reduces the production of prostaglandins and thromboxane, thereby decreasing pain.
- Platelet dysfunction, gastritis, and renal impairment are side effects that are dose dependent.
- There is controversy as to whether NSAIDs impair bone, tendon, and ligament healing.
  - This effect has been demonstrated in animal studies (based on histologic examination of the fracture healing site).
  - There are no human randomized controlled trials that have shown this effect.
  - Cohort studies have shown divergent effects and often factors such as the doses used and complicating factors such as smoking have not been described.
  - It is our recommendation that demonstrated analgesia benefit of NSAIDs outweighs the theoretical, but not demonstrated, risk of impaired healing.

Opioids

- Opioids are the mainstay of analgesia in the trauma setting.
- Intramuscular or subcutaneous administration of opioids is not recommended in a trauma setting as trauma patients will have highly variable tissue perfusion and drug delivery (and thus onset and duration) is unpredictable.
- For procedural pain (e.g., placement of a chest tube), short-acting pain medications such as fentanyl is recommended as the duration of action of the drug must parallel the relatively short duration of the procedure.
- Both visceral pain and opioids themselves may induce nausea. Concomitant treatment with anti-emetics should be considered.

Ketamine

- Provides analgesia and due to its sympathetic effects, it contributes to hemodynamic stability.
- It has been shown in sub-analgesic doses to synergistically improve fentanyl's efficacy.

- Research performed on ventilated patients in which CO_2 was monitored showed no increase in intracranial pressures when ketamine is used. Hence, the old doctor's myth about ketamine use and raised ICP should be discarded.
- Ketamine is a cardiac stimulant (via sympathetically mediated mechanisms), so its use in patients with cardiovascular disease is a possible problem as it can cause increased myocardial oxygen demand.
  - Pretreatment with benzodiazepines has been shown to reduce the cardiovascular effects of ketamine.

Special Populations

The Pregnant Trauma Patient

- NSAIDs
  - Salicylates in particular are trapped within the fetal circulation, due to the fetus' relatively higher pH.
  - The use of NSAIDS in the pregnant patient is not recommended due to adverse materno-fetal outcomes.
- Acetaminophen
  - First-line analgesic (and antipyretic) in the pregnant patient.
  - Assuming normal liver function, there is no dose adjustment required and the 4 g/24 hr ceiling is appropriate.
- Opioids
  - The primary concern with opioids in the pregnant patient relates to their use in the perinatal period.
  - Administration of opioids during labor may lead to neonatal respiratory and CNS depression.
  - Chronic high-dose use of opioids can induce an addiction/withdrawal syndrome in the neonate.

The Elderly Trauma Patient

- Elderly patients require careful monitoring, titration, and selection of medications due to the following:
  - Decreased drug metabolism and excretion due to age-related decline in renal and hepatic function.
  - Altered volume of distribution – they have relatively less lean muscle tissue and more fat.
  - Less cardiovascular and respiratory reserve.
    - Consequently, they are not as tolerant of cardiovascular and respiratory side-effects produced by analgesics, particularly opioid medications.
  - Due to the sympathetic drive induced by pain, they are more susceptible to cardiac demand ischemia in the setting of uncontrolled pain.
- Approach to pain control.
  - Start with lower doses of analgesics and then titrate to effect using additional, but relatively smaller doses of analgesics.

- For ongoing analgesia, use smaller doses and longer dosing intervals than you would in a younger patient.
- The elderly requires more frequent reassessment of pain and analgesic side effects compared to young patients.

The Pediatric Trauma Patient

- The basic neurological and hormone response to pain in the pediatric patient is effectively the same as in the adult patient.
  - Physiologic differences (see Chapters 13 and 22):
    - Neurological.
    - Relatively fewer inhibitory neurotransmitters in the spinal cord, which normally help to attenuate the perception of pain.
    - Less developed inhibitory synapses within the brain, which also help to attenuate the perception of pain.
- The clinical response to pain in the pediatric patient shows marked differences to the adult.
  - Neonates and infants exhibit a lower threshold to pain with repeated exposures as opposed to the habituation shown by adults.
  - Older children report increased perception of pain with repeated painful stimuli.
  - This is likely due to cognitive immaturity. Young children do not have the maturity to understand and differentiate the source and purpose of the painful stimulus. For example, the pain of the insertion of an IV to facilitate treatment compared to the pain of a fracture.
  - Oligo-analgesia has been associated with an increased development of PTSD in pediatric trauma patients.
- Drug metabolism considerations in children.
  - Hepatic metabolism
    - Liver becomes fully functional at 1 month of age.
    - At ages 2–6, the liver is relatively larger compared to the overall body mass, so drug metabolism is actually increased during this time period.
  - Renal metabolism
    - Renal blood flow, glomerular filtration, and tubular secretion are all reduced during the first year of life. Thus, renal excretion and metabolism of drugs is relatively reduced in the first year of life.
    - Renal function normalizes after the first year.
  - Drug distribution
    - Children have less body fat – lipid-soluble drugs are available in higher concentrations in the plasma.
    - Children have decreased protein binding – thus opioids and local anesthetics have relatively higher bioavailability in children.
- Recommendations in the pediatric trauma patient (see Chapters 13 and 22 for specific recommendations).
  - Assessing pain
    - Parental assessment of a child's pain should also be considered as they typically know their child the best.

- ▷ Clinical signs and symptoms of pain.
  - ○ Crying, grunting, and moaning. However, the pediatric patient may simply remain silent due to a fear of further injections.
  - ○ Tachycardia, hypertension, and tachypnea.
  - ○ Young children may exhibit a paradoxical vagal response to pain – bradycardia and attenuation of the normal sympathetic response. This is especially true in periods of prolonged pain.
  - ○ Increased muscle tone, agitation.
- ● Approach to treating pain
  - ▷ Evidence shows that pediatric trauma patients are consistently undertreated for pain due to fears of overdose.
  - ▷ If you are uncertain about the level of a child's pain, a trial of a small dose of analgesia is appropriate. Examine the child afterwards for objective evidence of any beneficial effect.
    - ○ Decrease in level of tachycardia, hypertension, and tachypnea.
    - ○ Decreased agitation and/or more interactive with you during the exam.
    - ○ Decreased muscle tone or voluntary guarding during the exam.
- ■ Pharmacologic approaches – see Chapter 22.

The Renal or Hepatic Failure Patient

- ■ Opioids are primarily metabolized by the liver and are renally excreted.
- ■ Hepatic failure
  - ● Begin with lower doses and longer dose intervals and titrate up, as opioids and benzodiazepines will terminate their action primarily by redistribution as opposed to metabolism.
  - ● Avoid morphine and codeine as these opioids have active metabolites. The ideal opioids in patients with hepatic failure are fentanyl and hydromorphone.
- ■ Renal failure
  - ● Morphine and codeine have active metabolites that are renally excreted, and thus will accumulate in the renal failure patient.
  - ● Fentanyl and hydromorphone are the ideal choices as they have inactive metabolites.

Specific Injuries and Specific Recommendations for Pain Control

Blunt Chest Trauma

- ■ Rib fractures
  - ● Systemic analgesia to prevent splinting and respiratory failure.
    - ▷ Achieve acute pain control with opioids.
    - ▷ Then give regular oral and/or IV analgesia.
    - ▷ Intercostal blocks or epidural analgesia is an option in the stable patient.

Extremity Fractures

- Splinting and casting
  - The definitive treatment for reducing the majority of the pain associated with a fracture.
- Elevation
- Hematoma block (see Chapter 12)
  - Most appropriate for Colles', Smith's, and metacarpal fractures.
- Peripheral nerve block (see Chapter 12)
  - Wrist block – phalangeal and metacarpal fractures, finger crush/amputation injuries.

Strains/Sprains

- Splinting/taping.
- Tensor bandage.
- NSAIDs and/or acetaminophen. Consider codeine.
- Walking aids – crutches may be necessary for brief period.

Burns

- Nonpharmacological methods:
  - If the burn is <30 minutes old, cooling the affected area with water (10–25 degrees celsius) helps to reduce the pain dramatically.
- Do not use ice as this will make the burn injury worse.
  - A moist dressing over the burn site is also effective.
  - Avoid air currents over the burn.
  - Avoid reinjury – heat sources or refreezing in the case of cold burns.
- Pharmacological methods:
  - For small area and relatively minor burns, simple oral analgesics such as acetaminophen or ibuprofen should be adequate. Consider codeine.
  - For large/severe burns in the acute setting, parenteral opioids are the most appropriate method of pain relief.
  - Intravenous lidocaine:
    - Mechanism of analgesia: inhibits neuronal activity of afferent neurons within the dorsal horn of the spinal cord.
    - A bolus dose of 1 mg/kg, then an infusion rate of 1–4 mg/min.
  - Benzodiazepines are useful in reducing the anxiety associated with the burn injury.
    - Remember that benzodiazepines and opioids have additive effects in causing respiratory depression and hypotension.

Suggested Reading

Atkinson P, et al. Pain management and sedation for children in the emergency department. Brit Med J 2009;339:1074–1079.

Buchimschi C, Weiner CP. Medications in pregnancy and lactation – part 2 drugs with minimal or unknown human teratogenic effect. Obstet Gynecol 2009;113 (2 Pt 1):417–432.

Cohen SP, Christo PJ, Moroz L. Pain Management in trauma patients. Am J Phys Med Rehabil 2004;83(2):142–161.

Curtis LA, Morrell TD. Pain management in the emergency department. Emerg Med Pract 2006;8(7):1–28.

Ferry ST, Dahners LE, Afshari HM, Weinhold PS. The effects of common anti-inflammatory drugs on the healing rat patellar tendon. Am J Sports Med 2007;35(8):1326.

Malchow RJ, Black IH. The evaluation of pain management in the critically ill trauma patient: Emerging concepts from the global war on terrorism. Crit Care Med 2008;36(7 Suppl):S346–S357.

Soloman DH. Overview of selective COX-2 inhibitor. UptoDate version 18.2, updated June 9, 2010.

Zatzick DF, Rivara FP, Nathens AB, et al. A nationwide U.S. study of post-traumatic stress after hospitalization for physical injury. Psychol Med 2007;37:1469–1480.

Zhang X, Schwarz EM, Young DA, Puzas JE, Rosier RN, O'Keefe RJ. Cyclooxygenase-2 regulates mesenchymal cell differentiation into the osteoblast lineage and is critically involved in bone repair. J Clin Invest 2002;109(11):1405.

21 Abdominal Pain

Sean Moore

Introduction

- Abdominal pain is the most common complaint in the emergency department (ED), accounting for one in nine patients who present.
- Most causes are benign and self-limiting, but approximately one in six may be serious or life threatening.
- Diagnosis is often difficult and may rely on elements from the patient demographics, history, past medical and surgical history, physical examination, laboratory tests, and imaging.
- The use of advanced medical imaging has increased significantly in recent years for patients with abdominal pain.
- In one-third of patients, a cause will not be found in the ED.
- The vast majority of patients with undifferentiated abdominal pain will improve spontaneously.
- Elderly patients are at high risk for serious and surgical pathologies.

Pathophysiology

- Abdominal pain is often approached anatomically, using the approximate location of the pain as a starting point.
- As innervation of organs and their capsules relates to their embryologic development or spinal nerve level, several organs may present with pain in similar areas.
- Symptoms may range from hypotension or shock, to nausea and vomiting, diarrhea, diffuse pain, anxiety, or localized pain depending on the organ affected.
- To differentiate the cause, it is essential to piece together elements from the history and physical examination to establish a pain pattern representative of more specific pathologies.
- Visceral pain is often described as deep, dull, and poorly localized.
  - It may be caused by distention, inflammation, or ischemic insults to organs.
  - Pain is often accompanied by anxiety, diaphoresis, or a feeling of impending doom.
    - The localization of pain is poor as pain fibers enter the spinal cord at multiple levels.

> ▶ Foregut organs, including the stomach, duodenum, liver, gallbladder, and pancreas produce upper abdominal pain.

> ▶ Midgut organs, including the small bowel, appendix, and proximal colon produce periumbilical pain.

> ▶ Hindgut structures, including the distal colon and the genitourinary system cause lower abdominal pain.

- Parietal pain or somatic abdominal pain is produced by ischemia, inflammation, or stretching of the parietal peritoneum.
  - Localization of pain is specific to the side and dermatome level of the pain, unlike visceral pain.
  - Pain is usually sharp, constant, and specific to the area of the organ in question.
- Referred pain is felt in an area distinct from the origin of pain.
  - It results from sharing of afferent neurons from different locations in the body.
  - Pain in non-abdominal areas may be referred to the abdomen. Examples include pneumonia, glaucoma, and myocardial infarction.
  - Pain derived from abdominal processes may be felt in other areas such as the pelvis or thorax. An example is biliary disease referred to the right shoulder.
  - No one description of abdominal pain can be definitively correlated with a specific cause.

Undifferentiated Abdominal Pain

- Those patients who are assessed to have nonsurgical abdominal examinations and are diagnosed with "undifferentiated abdominal pain" or abdominal pain NYD include approximately one-third of all cases of abdominal pain in the ED.
- The vast majority of patients leaving the ED will have complete resolution of pain within 2 weeks of discharge.
- Analgesia should be given at the earliest in patients with abdominal pain, including in those patients without a confirmed diagnosis.
- Withholding pain medication before diagnosis was based on antiquated methods, yet up to 76% of physicians fail to give appropriate analgesia for these patients prior to getting a surgical evaluation.
- Many studies show improved diagnostic accuracy when the patient is given analgesics.
- Those who receive opioids tend to have more severe disease and are associated with higher mortality, but no causal link has been established and analgesia should be viewed as an important aspect of care in the ED.
- Hemodynamically unstable patients need to have early aggressive supportive and surgical care prior to definitive diagnosis or imaging in many cases.

Abdominal Aortic Aneurysm

- Five percent of patients above 65 years have an abdominal aortic aneurysm (AAA).

- It is associated with atherosclerosis, smoking, hypertension, and family history.
- Ruptured AAA has a very high mortality. Early ED identification may decrease mortality from 75%–35%.
- Patients with AAA may present with severe abdominal, flank or back pain. This may be accompanied by radiation to the groin or thigh.
  - Occasionally, it may present with only syncope as the presenting complaint.
  - Syncope followed by abdominal pain or hypotension should be presumed to represent AAA until proven otherwise.
- Clinical examination may show hypotension, diffuse abdominal tenderness, pulsatile abdominal mass, abdominal bruits, abdominal or flank ecchymosis, or absent distal pulses.
- The triad of abdominal pain, hypotension, and a palpable pulsatile mass are seen in approximately one-half of patients with ruptured AAA.
- Clinical examination is of limited value and ultrasound (US) examination is recommended in the ED to rule in and rule out the disease.
  - US is 98% sensitive for detecting AAA.
  - US is much less reliable for detecting rupture.
  - A 5-cm AAA associated with abdominal pain is at imminent risk for rupture.
- Management:
  - Patients with hemodynamic instability and a history of AAA or have ED US confirmation of AAA need immediate surgical consultation and operative intervention.
  - Hypertensive patients with AAA should be treated with labetolol or esmolol when an expanding but unruptured AAA is associated with elevated blood pressure.
  - Analgesia should be given judiciously to avoid hypotension.
  - Angiography or CT may be used in stable patients after consultation with surgeon.
- Despite rapid management, patients have a high mortality from ruptured AAA, and 50% of those who survive to reach the operating room will die.

Appendicitis

- Appendicitis is the most common surgical cause of abdominal pain in adults.
- Appendicitis remains a difficult diagnosis, and missed diagnosis is one of the most common reasons for malpractice.
- It is challenging to diagnose in some cases, especially in pregnancy and elderly patients.
  - Only 20% of elderly patients present with classic symptoms of anorexia, fever, right lower quadrant (RLQ) pain, and leukocytosis.
- Typically presents as a poorly differentiated pain localizing to the periumbilical area, later localizing to the RLQ with peritoneal irritation. It is often associated with anorexia, fever, and nausea.
- Clinical examination may reveal tenderness in the RLQ, but may extend to anywhere along the length of the appendix.

- Examination may evolve to include peritoneal irritation with localized tenderness, and diffuse rigidity with increased irritation or perforation.
- The appendix may be located in several locations with relation to the cecum and may also extend past the midline and result in left lower quadrant (LLQ) pain.
- Laboratory findings:
  - High white blood cell (WBC) count may indicate a greater likelihood of appendicitis, but normal WBC is very common and does not exclude disease.
  - C-reactive protein (CRP) may similarly be elevated in acute appendicitis, but a normal CRP does not exclude disease.
- Imaging:
  - In typical presentations, patients may proceed to surgery without imaging.
  - CT or US imaging can help clarify the diagnosis.
  - Abdominal US is often chosen as first line to limit radiation in facilities with operators experienced in graded compression US.
  - CT scanning with or without contrast can be used to more reliably exclude the diagnosis in cases not confirmed by US.
  - Plain films are rarely helpful and not indicated.
- Serial examination should be done within 12 hours or earlier if symptoms evolve as longer delays may result in an increase in perforation.
- Management:
  - Generally, operative intervention with appendectomy is the accepted standard of care although antibiotics may be successful in eliminating some cases of appendicitis.
  - Antibiotics are used if there are signs of peritoneal irritation.
  - PiP-Taz 3.375 g IV or Cefoxitin 2 g IV Q6H are acceptable choices preoperatively.
- It is generally acceptable to operate within 12 hours of diagnosis.

Bowel Obstruction

- Bowel obstruction is the second most common cause for surgical intervention in the elderly.
- It may occur in small or large intestine.
  - Large-bowel obstruction may be caused by neoplasm, diverticulitis, or volvulus.
  - Small-bowel obstruction is most commonly caused by adhesions, hernias, or neoplasms.
- Causes may include extrinsic, intrinsic, or intraluminal processes.
  - Accumulation of gastric, biliary, pancreatic secretions, and oral intake.
  - Distention of bowels and perforation may occur.
  - Prior surgery may lead to adhesions, causing mechanical obstruction.
- Typically, pain is described as diffuse, poorly localized cramping and is moderate to severe.

■ Symptoms usually include:
  ● Nausea and vomiting.
  ● Bloating and inability to pass gas or stool.
  ● Abdominal distention.
■ Fever, general abdominal tenderness, peritoneal signs, and increased or high-pitched bowel sounds may be seen on examination.
■ Plain radiographs may show obstruction and remains one of the few clinical settings where plain films are used in workup of abdominal pain.
■ If obstruction is seen, most patients will require CT evaluation.

Diverticulitis

■ Typically in patients older than age 50.
■ Colonic diverticuli may become obstructed by fecal matter, resulting in bacterial growth and subsequent inflammation and distension.
■ Occurs in ~30% of patients with diverticulosis.
  ● Usually more common in sigmoid colon, thus presenting with left-sided pain.
  ● May occur anywhere throughout the colon.
  ● May occur in younger individuals who have more severe disease.
■ Typical presentation is fever, LLQ pain, and elevated WBC in a patient older than age 50.
  ● Patients may experience diarrhea or constipation.
  ● Nausea and vomiting may occur.
  ● Fifty percent of patients will have heme-positive stools.
  ● Patients may have toxic appearance if perforation has occurred.
■ Typically, pain is deep, unremitting, and may progress to severe diffuse pain if the patient has a perforation.
■ Palpation of a mass in the LLQ may be appreciated, and tenderness on rectal examination is common. A rigid abdomen with guarding may be present following perforation.
■ Imaging:
  ● CT is the test of choice for diverticulitis and the workup of undifferentiated abdominal pain in the elderly.
  ● Simple uncomplicated diverticulitis may be differentiated from abscessed or perforated diverticulitis on CT.
■ Management:
  ● Inpatient treatment involves analgesia, bowel rest, IV antibiotics, and surgical consultation.
  ● Outpatient treatment is appropriate for simple uncomplicated diverticulitis.
    ▶ Opioid analgesia.
    ▶ Bowel rest with clear fluids for 48 hours.
    ▶ Metronidazole 500 mg po TID plus Ciprofloxacin 500 mg po TID is an appropriate regimen for 10 days.
    ▶ Moxifloxacin 400 mg po OD for 10 days alternative.

Ectopic Pregnancy

- Ectopic pregnancy is the leading cause of pregnancy-related death.
- Ectopic implantation most commonly occurs in the distal ampulla of the fallopian tube.
- Forty percent are missed on the first ED visit.
- Two percent of all pregnancies are ectopic and the incidence is rising.
  - Risk increased with prior ectopic, IUD, PID, prior tube surgery, and assisted reproduction.
  - Over 50% of cases occur without any risk factors.
- Abdominal pain, missed menstrual period, and vaginal bleeding is the classic presentation, but is not reliably seen.
- All females of child-bearing age who present with abdominal pain need a pregnancy test.
- Pregnancy in a patient who has had prior tubal ligation should be considered ectopic until proven otherwise.
- Clinical examination is not reliable in excluding ectopic pregnancy.
  - Patients may be hemodynamically unstable or stable following rupture.
  - Uterine size is often the same as intrauterine pregnancies.
- Serum quantitative HCG testing may show failure to double in 48 hours.
  - An increase of <50% in 48 hours indicates an abnormal pregnancy.
  - Transvaginal US should show an intrauterine pregnancy (IUP) by the time the HCG is >1,500 mIU/mL.
  - Transabdominal US should show an IUP by the time the HCG is >5,000.
  - HCG <1,000 does *not* preclude US utility.
  - Thirty percent of ectopics are seen with HCG readings below 1,000.
- US should be done in the ED to assess for free fluid and IUP.
- Patients with free fluid and no IUP should obtain emergent surgical consultation for operative intervention.
- Management:
  - Medical management:
    - Methotrexate is used only in reliable patients who are hemodynamically stable with small ectopic pregnancy (<4 cm), HCG < 5,000 and no free fluid on US.
    - Contraindications include hepatic or renal dysfunction, blood dyscrasia, impaired immune function, and breastfeeding.
    - Methotrexate should be offered after consultation with gynecology.
- Surgical management:
  - Surgical treatment with laparotomy and salpingostomy or salpingectomy is the treatment of choice in unstable patients.
- Pearls:
  - Twenty percent of women with abdominal pain and bleeding in the first trimester will have an ectopic pregnancy.
  - Twenty percent of ruptured ectopic pregnancies will have normal vital signs despite class IV shock.

Epiploic Appendigitis

- Epiploic appendigitis is much more commonly diagnosed with the increased use of CT and US scanning in abdominal pain.
- Typically seen in young adults and may be seen in the LLQ or less commonly in the RLQ.
- Diarrhea may be seen in 25% of cases.
- The colon typically has approximately 50–100 fatty appendinges, which may become torsed, resulting in necrosed tissue and surrounding inflammation.
- Examination may reveal focal tenderness, usually in the LLQ.
- Guarding and rebound tenderness may occur with local peritoneal irritation.
- Management:
  - This disease process is self-limiting and does not require antibiotics for treatment.
  - Nonsteroidal anti-inflammatory drugs (NSAIDs) may reduce the pain of epiploic appendigitis.
  - Opioid analgesics should be provided for pain control.

GI Bleeds/Peptic Ulcer Disease

- Most peptic ulcers are now knows to be caused by *H. pylori* infection.
- It is classically described as burning epigastric pain but may be sharp, dull or aching. The pain may be relieved by eating and awaken the patient from sleep.
  - Rapid change in typical pain may represent perforation. Will usually have associated hemodynamic instability.
  - New onset of back pain in a patient with peptic ulcer disease (PUD) may represent ulceration into the pancreas with associated pancreatitis.
- Pearl: 50% of elderly patients with PUD present with acute abdomen.
- Nausea, coffee ground emesis, or vomiting blood may be associated or independent of pain.
- Melena stools may be seen in upper GI bleeds, and stools with bright red blood may also occur in larger bleeds or those with rapid passage of blood through the GI tract.
- Investigations:
  - CBC, liver function testing, lipase, and blood type for cross-match should be obtained early.
  - Radiographs may show free air below the diaphragm.
  - CT may help clarify the diagnosis in patients with peritonitis of unclear etiology.
- Management:
  - Patients should be kept NPO.
  - Supportive care should include aggressive fluid management and early blood administration in unstable patients.
  - Proton pump inhibitors such as pantoprazole 80 mg bolus followed by 8 mg/hr drip helps raise the gastric pH rapidly.

- Broad-spectrum antibiotics are recommended when complicated by perforation.
- Admission and surgical consultation should be obtained for patients with hemorrhage, perforation, or obstruction.

Hernias

- Hernias result from a defect in the abdominal wall. Abdominal contents, including fat, peritoneum, omentum, or abdominal organs, may pass through the defect transiently or become incarcerated or strangulated.
- Pain is usually localized to the area of the hernia.
  - Most commonly hernias are in the inguinal area.
  - There may be a history of heavy lifting.
  - Femoral hernias are more commonly seen in females.
  - Incisional, abdominal wall, and periumbilical hernias are also possible.
- Fever and tachycardia may be present with irreducible hernias.
- Hernias that are not incarcerated may be reproduced by increasing intra-abdominal pressure.
- Investigations:
  - WBC may be elevated, but is not reliable finding.
  - Plain films may show perforation if the incarceration has resulted in perforation.
  - US or CT may be useful in confirming the diagnosis.
- Management:
  - Reduction may be attempted manually, but often requires emergent surgical intervention.
  - In cases where there is question of delayed presentation where necrotic bowel may be present, manual reduction is not advisable.
  - Patients should be kept NPO and IV hydration started pending surgical consultation.
  - Opioid analgesia should be offered.

Inflammatory Bowel Disease

- Inflammatory bowel disease (IBD) is a chronic disease characterized by intermittent exacerbation of abdominal pain.
- It is often subdivided into Crohn's, ulcerative colitis, and indeterminate colitis.
- Clinical features of the disease are often related to the anatomic distribution and severity of disease.
  - Abdominal pain is often severe. It may be crampy, colicky, or unrelenting.
  - Bloody diarrhea, weight loss, and anorexia are commonly seen but symptoms are highly individualized.
  - Fever and toxicity may be present in cases complicated by abscess.
  - Extraintestinal manifestations include arthritis, episcleritis, uveitis, erythema nodosum, hepatobiliary disease, renal colic, and thromboembolic complications.

- The course is unpredictable, but flare ups and remissions are highly individualized.
- Examination may reveal diffuse or localized tenderness depending on the individual.
- Laboratory tests may include CBC, electrolytes, CRP, and occasionally type and cross-match.
- CT imaging may be indicated to assess surgical pathology if complications are suspected.
- Management:
  - Analgesia in these patients is challenging as patients with chronic pain require high doses of opioids.
    - Many patients are inappropriately labeled as drug seekers.
    - Patients with pseudo-addiction may normalize when pain is appropriately treated.
    - Chronic pain results in complex psychosocial adaptation and patients may be challenging for many physicians.
    - Parental opioids are normally needed for pain in IBD.
  - Consultation with gastroenterology or surgery is indicated for patients who have significant complications, treatment failure, or peritoneal signs.
  - Mainstays of treatment include steroids, antibiotics for abscesses, immunosuppressive drugs, 5-ASA preparations, immune modulators, and surgical intervention.
  - Hydration, analgesia, and serial examination should be done within 12 hours or earlier if symptoms evolve as longer delays may result in an increase in perforation.
- Complications may include abscess, fissure, fistulas, rectal prolapsed, malnutrition, and malabsorption.

Mesenteric Ischemia

- Mesenteric ischemia is usually divided into arterial or venous disease.
  - Arterial mesenteric ischemia is divided into low flow states and occlusive disease.
  - Occlusive disease is subdivided into thrombotic or embolic.
- Pain may be gradual onset (low flow) or acute (embolism).
- Pain tends to be poorly localized and dull but may be out of proportion to clinical findings.
- Pearl: Pain out of proportion to examination is a very worrisome finding.
- The patient may have significant nausea and vomiting.
- Patients may feel significant anxiety, impending doom, or appear relatively well, making the diagnosis very difficult.
- Patients later in presentation may have a toxic appearance with hypotension and instability.
- Serum lactate rises late in the disease process and is a poor prognostic sign.
- Radiography or CT may show pneumatosis intestinalis or portal vein gas.
  - May get false reassurance of alternate diagnosis if ileus or obstruction is found.

- Angiography, CT, or MRI may be used, but none is completely reliable for detecting mesenteric ischemia.
- Despite aggressive treatment, surgical intervention to remove necrotic bowel, and supportive care, survival is 50% when diagnosed within 24 hours.

Ovarian Torsion

- Ovarian or adnexal torsion occurs when the ovary or fallopian tube twists and cuts off its blood supply.
- Early diagnosis and surgical treatment are essential if fertility is to be preserved.
- It can occur at any age but primarily in reproductive years, with 20% occurring during pregnancy.
- Pain is typically sudden onset and located in the lower abdomen and pelvis. It localizes to the affected side, and is sharp and severe in nature.
- Radiation of the pain may be to the back, pelvis, or groin.
- Late presentations may be associated with fever, peritonitis, or sepsis.
- The ovary will remain viable for approximately 6 hours from the time of torsion.
- Ninety-five percent of torsion occurs in abnormal adnexa (examples include tumors or cysts).
- US with color flow assessment of blood flow is the test of choice for diagnosis.
- Management:
  - Consult gynecology for surgical management.

Pancreatitis

- Pancreatitis typically presents as severe dull epigastric pain, which may radiate through to the back. Severe cases may be associated with hemodynamic instability.
- Patients typically have local tenderness in the epigastric area.
- Investigations:
  - Workup should include electrolytes, lipase, and contrast abdominal CT.
    - Lipase may be elevated in alcoholic patients in absence of pancreatitis.
  - CT can be used to assess complications such as pseudocyst, abscess, and can grade severity, which helps with prognostication.
  - If a biliary cause is suspected, US may be performed to assess mechanical common bile duct obstruction. ERCP or MRCP may be needed in some cases.
- Management involves aggressive supportive care.
- IV fluids.
- Analgesia.
- Keep patient NPO.
- Medical versus surgical consultation will depend on the cause of pancreatitis.

Pelvic Inflammatory Disease

- Pelvic inflammatory disease is an infection of the female reproductive tract caused by ascending sexually transmitted infection from the vagina or cervix.

- It is the single most common serious infection in women of child-bearing age and affects one million Americans yearly.
- Two-thirds of cases go unrecognized, and may lead to serious sequelae including peritonitis, chronic pelvic pain, infertility, and increased risk for ectopic pregnancy.
- Up to 15% of affected women will become infertile after infection.
- PID is commonly caused by *Chlamydia trachomatis and Neisseria gonorrheae,* with many patients suffering from polymicrobial infections.
- Lower abdominal or pelvic pain is the most common presentation. Pain may be associated with vaginal discharge, bleeding, dysuria, or dyspareunia.
- CDC criteria for PID includes:
  - Major criteria (should all be present):
    - Cervical motion tenderness.
    - Lower abdominal tenderness.
    - Adnexal tenderness.
  - Minor criteria (may help to enhance specificity):
    - Temperature >38°C.
    - Abnormal vaginal or cervical discharge.
    - Elevated ESR or CRP.
    - Documented gonorrhea or *Chlamydia* infection.
    - Used in daily practice.
- US may be used to assess tubo-ovarian abscess.
  - It may also show alternate diagnosis such as appendicitis or ovarian torsion.
  - Does not exclude disease, as PID is a clinical diagnosis.
- If no other cause of lower abdominal pain or tenderness is found, it is advisable to treat as PID in the absence of formal criteria as missed disease can result in serious consequences and complications.
- Management:
  - Patients need to be hospitalized if the patient is not responding to oral therapy, cannot tolerate oral treatment, has fever, there is evidence of tubo-ovarian abscess, or other surgical diagnosis cannot be excluded.
  - Intravenous antibiotic regimens may include doxycycline 100 mg IV/po BID plus cefoxitin 2 g IV Q6H.
  - Outpatient regimens may include ceftriaxone 250 mg IM plus doxycycline 100 mg po BID for 14 days plus metronidazole 500 mg po BID for 14 days (CDC guidelines 2010).
  - Supportive therapy should include intravenous fluids, analgesia, and anti-nausea medications.
  - Opioid analgesia and NSAIDs may be used to treat associated pelvic pain.

Testicular Torsion

- The incidence of torsion is 1 in 4,000 and often occurs in young males.
- Torsion of the testis results from twisting of the testes when there is abnormal fixation of the testis within the tunica vaginalis.

- Typically, pain is acute lower abdominal, pelvic, groin, or testicular pain. The pain may be constant or intermittent.
  - Associated nausea and vomiting is common.
  - Abdominal pain is the presenting complaint in 20%.
- It is essential to examine the testes in all males with abdominal pain.
  - The testis may be firm, tender, and at a higher and transverse lie.
- Laboratory and urine testing are not helpful.
- Doppler US may be used if the diagnosis is in doubt.
- Management:
  - Emergent surgery is essential to preserve viability of the testis.
  - Surgical exploration is gold standard for diagnosis and delay for testing should be avoided.
  - Manual detorsion should be attempted preoperatively if there is any delay to the OR.
    - Detorsion of the affected testis is performed by rotating the testis in a manner similar to opening a book when viewing the testes from the patient's feet. Relief of pain is a positive end point.
  - Eighty to 100% testicle viability if OR within 6 hours, but drops to 20% at 10 hours.

Volvulus

- Volvulus may occur in the stomach, cecum, colon, or sigmoid.
- Commonly volvulus may be associated with chronic constipation.
- Volvulus typically presents as crampy lower abdominal pain.
- Physical examination typically reveals diffuse tenderness and abdominal distension.
- Laboratory testing should include CBC, electrolytes, renal function, and lactate.
- Imaging:
  - Plain films may be diagnostic.
  - CT is often necessary to elucidate any underlying volvulus may occur in the stomach, cecum, colon, or sigmoid.
- Management:
  - Volvulus is a surgical disease and requires early intervention.
  - Supportive care and fluid replacement should be prompt.
  - Broad-spectrum antibiotic administration such as Pip-Taz 3.375 mg IV Q6H should be given to patients.

Abdominal Pain in Women of Child-Bearing Age

- Abdominal pain in women of child-bearing age range from benign to life-threatening etiologies including ectopic pregnancy, PID, adnexal torsion, ovarian cyst, endometriosis, fibroids, appendicitis, renal colic, and biliary disease.
- *All* women of child-bearing age need a pregnancy test.

- History must include menstrual history, sexual history, and any genitourinary symptoms.
- Examination should routinely include pelvic examination.
- Urinalysis with HCG is essential to direct the further care.
  - Positive HCG testing should be followed with quantitative testing.
- CBC is routinely obtained, but may not be helpful in diagnosis.
- A blood type/cross-match should be available for all women of child-bearing age who are pregnant and experiencing abdominal pain or are hemodynamically unstable.
- US is generally the imaging test of choice in pregnancy to avoid radiation.
- Analgesia should be given to treat painful conditions, keeping in mind potential that patients may be pregnant.
- PID is the most common serious infection among reproductive age women.
  - Majority of PID goes unrecognized.
  - Must be vigilant in looking for PID as complications are serious and may include infertility or increased risk of ectopic pregnancy.

Abdominal Pain in the Elderly

- Age in years roughly equals the probability of admission.
- Elderly patients are at higher risk for inadequate analgesia.
- These patients are also at higher risk for adverse reactions and interactions with opioids, and smaller doses should be used while titrating accordingly.
- High risk for serious pathology such as AAA, ischemic bowel, myocardial infarction, and perforated bowel.
- Most common diagnoses are biliary disease, undifferentiated abdominal pain, appendicitis bowel obstruction, and diverticulitis. Delayed diagnosis is very common.
- Mortality is markedly higher and patients may have more rapid progression of disease in the elderly population.
  - Overall mortality is ~10%.
- Diagnosis is generally more difficult with increasing age.
  - Presenting complaints and physical examination accuracy are much less reliable with advancing age.
- Laboratory testing is usually indicated, but may be misleading.
  - Normal WBC is seen in many patients with advanced surgical diagnosis.
  - Serum lactate and blood gases may be useful in identifying underappreciated serious pathology, but generally only appears late in processes such as mesenteric ischemia.
  - Lipase and liver function testing may also be inaccurate but can be useful.
- Advanced imaging is generally indicated for elderly patients with abdominal pain complaints.
  - ED US is an important consideration for patients with possible AAA.
- Serial examination and admission should be the norm for elderly patients without clear diagnosis.

Abdominal Pain in Immunocompromised and HIV

- Patients with altered immunity may develop unusual conditions including drug-induced pancreatitis, antiretroviral-induced lactic acidosis, AIDS-cholangiopathy, bacterial colitis, typhilitis, or other opportunistic infections.
- Abdominal pain is related to immune dysfunction in ~65% of AIDS patients.
  - Patients may have the usual pathologies seen by other populations as well.
- Causes may include lymphoma, CMV esophagitis/gastritis/enteritis, colitis, sclerosing cholangitis, and cryptosporidial infection.
- Clinical examination alone is rarely diagnostic in this group.
- Correlation of CD4 count may be helpful when considering opportunistic infections.
- Advanced imaging is usually indicated in patients with HIV and abdominal pain as serious pathology is common and may not be clinically apparent.

Summary

- Abdominal pain is a common presentation to the ED with a variety of causes.
- Several life-threatening causes need emergent investigations and specific treatment.

Suggested Reading

American College of Emergency Physicians. Critical issues in the evaluation and management of emergency department patients with suspected appendicitis. Ann Emerg Med 2010;55:71–116.

American College of Obstetricians and Gynecologists Practice Bulletin No 94. Medical management of ectopic pregnancy. Obstet Gynecol 2008;111(6):1479–1485.

Bhuiya F, Pitts SR, McCaig LF. Emergency department visits for chest pain and abdominal pain: United States, 1999–2008. NCHS data brief, no 43. Hyattsville, MD: National Center for Health Statistics, 2010.

Cardall T, Glasser J, Guss DA. Clinical value of the total white blood cell count and temperature in the evaluation of patients with suspected appendicitis. Acad Emerg Med 2004;11:1021–1027.

Ciccone A, Allegra JR, Cochrane DG, et al. Age related differences in diagnoses with the elderly population. Am J Emerg Med 1998;157:276–280.

Hendrickson M, Naparst TR. Abdominal surgical emergencies in the elderly. Emerg Med Clin North Am 2003;21:937–969.

Kachalia A, Gandhi TK, Puopolo AL, et al. Missed and delayed diagnoses in the emergency department: a study of closed malpractice claims from 4 liability insurers. Ann Emerg Med 2007;49:196–205.

Karkhanis S, Medcalf J. Plain abdomen radiographs: the right view? Eur J Emerg Med 2009;16(5):267–270.

Lee JS, Stiell IG, Wells GA, et al. Adverse outcomes and opioid analgesic administration in acute abdominal pain. Acad Emerg Med 2000;7(9):980–987.

Lukens TW, Emerman C, Effron D. The natural history and clinical findings in undifferentiated abdominal pain. Ann Emerg Med 1993;22(4):690–696.

Oldenburg WA, Lau LL, Rodenberg TJ, et al. Acute mesenteric ischemia. Arch Intern Med 2004;164(10):1054–1062.

Pietrow PK, Karellas ME. Medical management of common urinary calculi. Am Fam Physician 2006;74(1):86–94.

Rosenstein D, McAninch JW. Urologic emergencies. Med Clin North Am 2004;88: 495–518.

Singh A, Alter H, Littlepage A. A systematic review of medical therapy to facilitate passage of ureteral calculi. Ann Emerg Med 2007;50:552–563.

Teichman JM. Clinical practice. Acute renal colic from ureteral calculus. N Engl J Med. 2004;350(7):684–693.

Thomas SH, et al. Effects of morphine analgesia on diagnostic accuracy in emergency department patients with abdominal pain: a prospective, randomized trial. J Am Coll Surg 2003;196(1):18–31.

van Geloven AA, Biesheuvel TH, Luitse JS, et al. Hospital admissions of patients aged over 80 with acute abdominal complaints. Eur J Surg 2000;166:866–871.

Wolfe JM, Lein DY, Lenkoski K, et al. Analgesic administration to patients with an acute abdomen: A survey of emergency medicine physicians. Am J Emerg Med 2000;18(3):250–253.

Wolfe JM, Smithline HA, Phipen S, et al. Does morphine change the physical examination in patients with acute appendicitis? Am J Emerg Med 2004;22(4):280–285.

Worster A, Richards C. Fluids and diuretics for acute ureteric colic. Cochrane Database Syst Rev 2005;(3):CD004926.

22 Pediatric Pain Management

Suzan Schneeweiss

Introduction

- There is a lack of recognition and treatment of pain in children.
- Pain relief for adult patients in the emergency department (ED) is 73% versus 53% for children.
  - Younger preverbal children generally receive less analgesics than older children.
- Medical procedures in the ED are often painful, unexpected, and heightened by stress and anxiety.
- Use of analgesic agents allows child to be more comfortable and improves cooperation during diagnostic evaluation.
- Appropriate management of pain reduces negative long-term effects of pain which include:
  - Conditioned anxiety response.
  - Increased response to pain with subsequent procedures.
  - Diminished analgesic response at subsequent visit.
  - "Blood-injection-injury phobia," which affects up to 25% of adult population.

Pain Assessment

- See Chapter 13.
- Need to consider the following with a careful pain assessment:
  - Age of child.
  - Developmental level.
  - Cognitive and communication skills.
  - Previous pain experiences.
  - Associated beliefs.
- Pain history: location, intensity, quality, duration, frequency, duration, and aggravating and relieving factors.
- Pain assessment and documentation improves administration of analgesics.

Three Main Methods Are Currently Used to Measure Pain Intensity

- Self-report – considered gold standard.

- Behavioral measures
  - Crying, facial expressions, body postures, and movements.
  - Generally used with neonates, infants, and younger children where communication is difficult.
- Physiologic measures
  - Heart rate, blood pressure, respiration, oxygen saturation, palmer sweating, and sometimes neuroendocrine responses.
  - Similar physiological responses occur during stress, which result in difficulty distinguishing stress versus pain responses.

Developmental Issues

- Children have pain words by 18–24 months (e.g., "hurt," "ow," "ouch").
- Word "pain" appears much later in children's vocabularies.
- Children can report degree of pain by 3–4 years.
- Children >6 years can provide detailed descriptions of pain intensity, quality, and location.

Pain Scales (See Chapter 13)

FLACC (Face, Legs, Activity, Cry, Consolability)

- For infants and children ages 2 months–7 years and cognitively impaired.
- See Table 22.1.

TABLE 22.1: FLACC scale for pain assessment

Category	0	1	2
Face	No particular expression or smile	Occasional grimace or frown, withdrawn, disinterested	Frequent to constant quivering chin, clenched jaw
Legs	Normal position or relaxed	Uneasy, restless, tense	Kicking, or legs drawn up
Activity	Lying quietly, normal position, moves easily	Squirming, shifting back and forth, tense	Arching, rigid or jerking
Cry	No cry (awake or asleep)	Moans or whimpers; occasional complaint	Crying steadily, screams or sobs, frequent complaints
Consolability	Content, relaxed	Reassured by occasional touching, hugging, or being talked to, distractible	Difficult to console or comfort

Each of the five categories is scored from 0–2, which results in a total score of 0–10.
From Merkel SI, Voepel-Lewis T, Shayevitz JR, Malyvia S. The FLACC: a behavioral scale for scoring postoperative pain in young children. Pediatr Nurs 1997;23(3):293–297.

Pain Word Scale

▪ For children ages 3–7 years and older children unable to use numerical rating scale.

▪ "None," "a little," "medium," and "a lot."

Faces Pain Scale-Revised (FPS-R)

▪ For ages 5–12 years (Figure 22.1).

   ● Point to the face that shows how much you hurt. Score the chosen face 0, 2, 4, 6, 8, or 10, so "0" = no pain and "10" = very much pain.

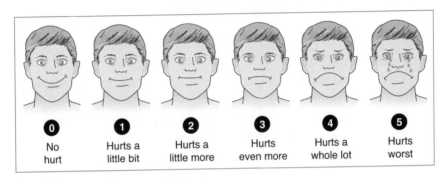

0	1	2	3	4	5
No hurt	Hurts a little bit	Hurts a little more	Hurts even more	Hurts a whole lot	Hurts worst

FIGURE 22.1: Faces scale for pain assessment.

Numerical Rating Scale

▪ For children >7 years.

▪ Numerical scales from 0–10 or 0–100.

Nonpharmacologic Measures for Pain Management

▪ See Chapter 13.

▪ Neonates and Infants:

   ● Nonnutritive sucking.

   ● Skin to skin contact with the mother (kangaroo care).

   ● Rocking and holding the infant.

   ● Swaddling the infant.

▪ Toddlers and preschoolers

   ● Active distraction: blowing bubbles, providing toys with lots of colors or toys that light up, distracting conservations.

   ● Passive distraction: reading age-appropriate book to child, singing songs, and practicing "blowing out birthday candles."

▪ Child

   ● Active techniques: blowing bubbles, singing songs, using squeeze balls, relaxation breathing, and playing with electronic devices.

   ● Passive distraction: watching videos, listening to music on headphones, reading a book to the child, or telling them a story.

- Adolescent
  - Ensure private setting.
  - Allow to choose method of distraction, presence of friends/family.
  - Active distraction: striking conversation, using squeeze balls, and playing with electronic devices.
  - Passive distraction: watching videos, training them to breathe deeply (in from the nose, count to 5 and out through the mouth), and listening to music.

Pharmacological Measure for Pain Management

Guidelines for Pain Management

- Prevent pain whenever possible; lower analgesic requirements with pretreatment for painful procedures.
- Adequate assessment of pain is key to appropriate management of pain.
- Give analgesics regularly.
- Use least invasive route; avoid IM injections whenever possible.
- Use WHO pain analgesic ladder (see Figure 22.2).
  - Match analgesic to pain severity.
  - Use more than one class of analgesics to promote better pain relief and reduce opioid requirement.

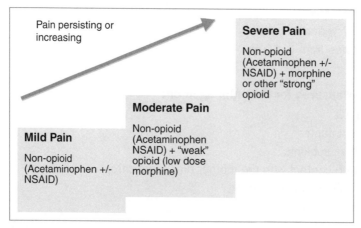

FIGURE 22.2: WHO pain analgesic ladder.

Non-opioid Analgesics

- See Table 22.2.

Acetaminophen

- Do not exceed maximum daily recommended dose of 75 mg/kg/day or 4 g/day if >12 years.
- Avoid using combination of opioid-acetaminophen (e.g., Tylenol #3) products as it is difficult to titrate.

TABLE 22.2: Analgesics for mild pain in pediatric patients

Analgesic	Dosage	Advantages	Disadvantages
Acetaminophen Drops: 80 mg/mL Suspension: 32 mg/mL Chewtab: 80 mg Suppositories: 120, 325, 650 mg, respectively	10–15 mg/kg q4–6 hr po 10–20 mg/kg PR Dose limit: 75 mg/kg/day or 4 g/d if >12 yrs, whichever is less	Well tolerated Safe	Liver toxicity if overdosed
Ibuprophen Drops: 40 mg/mL Suspension: 20 mg/mL	5–10 mg/kg po q6–8 hr Dose limit: 40 mg/kg/d or 2,400 mg/d adult	Longer duration of action	Gastrointestinal (GI) irritation Increased risk of bleeding after tonsillectomy
Naproxen Suspension: 25 mg/mL Tablets: 125, 250, 375 mg, respectively	10–20 mg/kg/d po divided bid Dose limit 1 g/d	Long duration of action Oral suspension	GI irritation

GI, gastrointestinal.

Nonsteroidal Anti-inflammatory Drugs

- Nonsteroidal anti-inflammatory drugs (NSAIDs) have a ceiling effect after which there is no additional analgesic benefit when maximum dose of an NSAID is attained.
- All NSAIDs offer same degree of analgesic effect (e.g., no advantage of IV ketorolac vs. po ibuprophen).
- Controversy regarding use of NSAIDs for fractures.
  - Affect bone healing in animal models, but this has not been shown in humans.
- Avoid NSAIDs for children with suspected or known inflammatory bowel disease and renal disease.

Sucrose (24% Solution)

- Effective method of procedural analgesia in neonates and young infants <6 months.
- Combine with other nonpharmacologic methods and pharmacologic measures.
- *Indications:* procedural pain including venipuncture, heel sticks, catheter insertion, LP, suturing, dressing changes, injections, and IV starts.
- One to 2 mL dripped onto anterior portion of tongue 2 minutes prior to procedure (maximum daily dose: 4 times in 24 hours).
- Increase efficacy when used with pacifier.

Opioid Analgesics

- See Table 22.3.
- Opioids are the most widely used agents for moderate to severe pain.

TABLE 22.3: Analgesics for moderate to severe pain in pediatric patients

Analgesic	Dosage	Advantages	Disadvantages
Morphine	**Intermittent dosing:** 0.2–0.4 mg/kg po/PR q4 hr child >50 kg 10–20 mg q3–4 hr 0.05–0.1 mg/kg IV/subcut q2–4 hr Dose limit: 15 mg/dose IV/subcut **Continuous infusion:** 0.1–0.2 mg/kg loading dose 0.01–0.04 mg/kg/hr IV/subcut infusion	Oral morphine more palatable than oral codeine, less GI effects Rapid onset Potent, analgesic	Respiratory depression Hypotension
Codeine	0.5–1 mg/kg po/IM q4–6 hr Maximum 1.5 mg/kg/dose 6 mg/kg/d (120 mg) Usual adult dose: 30–60 mg/dose	Potent analgesic No renal or hepatic toxicity Low addiction potential	Nausea Constipation Variability in metabolism to morphine (consider oral morphine)
Fentanyl	0.5–2.0 mcg/kg IV 1.4 mcg/kg Intranasal	Potent analgesic Less hypotension	Respiratory depression Apnea, chest wall rigidity
Hydromorphone	Intermittent IV: 0.015–0.02 mg/kg/ dose q2–4 hr Dose limit: 0.2–0.6 mg/dose IV Continuous infusion: 4–8 mcg/kg/hr IV Children ≤50 kg: 0.04–0.08 mg/kg/ dose po q3–4 hr prn Children >50 kg: 2–4 mg/ dose po q3–4 hr prn	Potent analgesic Alternative to morphine	Respiratory depression Hypotension

GI, gastrointestinal.

- They have no ceiling effect.
  - Increasing dose generates more analgesic effect (titrate the dose to pain intensity), but also increases risk of adverse effects.
  - Therefore, appropriate monitoring is necessary.
- Treating pain with opioid analgesics does not lead to psychological dependence or addiction.

Codeine

- Weak opiate; good analgesic for moderate pain.
- Combined tablets with acetaminophen limits flexibility in dosing, therefore best prescribed separately in pediatrics.
- Analgesic effect dependent on metabolism to morphine.
  - Codeine is metabolized to morphine by cytochrome p450 enzyme CYP2D6.
  - Genetic variability of enzyme activity with a significant number of poor metabolizers or non-metabolizers, and extensive metabolizers – patients in whom this medication will not work well.
  - Less reliable and efficacious than morphine.

Morphine

- Gold standard.
- Half-life of morphine varies with age.
  - Nine hours in preterm neonates, 6.5 hours in term neonates, and 2 hours in older infants and children.
- Delayed renal clearance of morphine metabolites may contribute to the analgesic, respiratory depressant, and rarely convulsant effects of morphine in the neonate.
- Induces histamine release (cautious use in patients with asthma and hypovolemia).

Hydromorphone

- Derivative of morphine (five to seven times more potent than morphine).
- Causes less sedation, pruritus, and nausea than morphine.
- Useful alternative to parenteral morphine.

Fentanyl

- Eighty to 100 times more potent than morphine.
- Few cardiovascular effects other than bradycardia; ideal in patients with congenital heart disease and trauma (neurosurgical) victims.
- Ideal for procedures as has a short duration of action (<60 minutes).
- Chest wall and glottic rigidity are complications to be monitored carefully.
  - Generally tends to occur with high (>5 mcg/kg) bolus but may occur even with low doses (1–2 mcg/kg).
  - Treated with naloxone or neuromuscular blockade and controlled mechanical ventilation.
- *Intranasal fentanyl* allows painless administration of analgesia, equivalent to IV morphine for pain.
  - Onset of action 4 minutes.
  - No serious adverse effects.
  - Equivalent to IV morphine for pain.
  - Patient positioning – sitting at 45-degree angle; use nasal atomizer device for improved drug delivery.
  - Maximum volume for nasal administration, generally 1 mL.

Management of Procedural Pain

- Ensure child-center approach (listen to needs of child and family) (see Chapter 13).
- Use parents for positive assistants rather than negative restraint.
- Active participation of child and family as opposed to passive recipients.
- Use least invasive equipment where possible.
- Use appropriate combination of nonpharmacologic and pharmacologic interventions.

- Sedation alone does not provide pain relief.
- Ensure that procedures are carried out to maximize patient safety.
- The following should be addressed prior to any procedure:
  - Explanation of need and importance of procedure.
  - An accurate description of the procedure.
  - Expectation of the intensity and duration of pain the child may experience.
  - Possible need for repeated procedural attempts.
  - Measures used to alleviate pain.
  - Parental guidance as to how child may react to pain.

Local Anesthesia

- Needle injection, venipuncture, and IV cannulation are common procedures in the pediatric ED, but may cause significant pain and anxiety.
- Consider the following strategies:

Strategies to Reduce Pain with Injection

- Use a small, long needle (30 G).
- Consider distraction techniques.
- Inject slowly.
- Buffered solution: add 1 mL $NaHCO_3$ to 9 mL lidocaine solution.
  - Neutralizes pH of lidocaine without affecting analgesic properties.
  - Stable at room temperature for 1 week.
- J-tip syringe
  - Sterile, single-use, needle-less syringe that delivers medication under high pressure from a compressed carbon dioxide gas cartridge.
  - Used for injection of buffered lidocaine for intravenous cannulation.
  - Medication penetrates to depth of 5–8 mm in 0.2 seconds.
  - Found to be more effective than EMLA® and Maxilene® in reducing pain with IV cannulation.

Topical Anesthetics for Intact Skin

- See Table 22.4.
- Can be used safely in neonates.
- Be cautions with the use of EMLA® in neonates as it can result in methemoglobinemia. Risk factors include reduced level of methemoglobin reductase, prolonged exposure/repeat use, and using other methemoglobin-inducing agents concurrently.
  - Can cause methemoglobinemia.
- EMLA® is less effective than oral glucose solution for venipuncture/heel prick.

TABLE 22.4: Comparison of different topical analgesic agents

	EMLA™	AMETOP™	MAXILENE™
Pharmacology	Eutectic mixture of two amide-type local anesthetics, lidocaine, and prilocaine	4% tetracaine, ester anesthetic	4% liposome encapsulated lidocaine
Onset of action	60 min with vaso-occlusive dressing to intact skin	30–45 min with vaso-occlusive dressing to intact skin	30 min with or without vaso-occlusive dressing
Duration of action	1–2 hrs	Up to 4–6 hrs	1–2 hrs
Contraindications	Hypersensitivity to amide type anesthetics Congenital or idiopathic methemoglobinemia Children 6–12 mo receiving sulphonamides	Hypersensitivity to ester-type local anesthetics, PABA Patients with low plasma cholinesterase	Hypersensitivity to amide-type local anesthetics Avoid near mucous membranes
Adverse effects	Local reactions: whitening or erythema, slight edema, burning, or itching	Local reactions: slight erythema, slight edema, pruritus Contact sensitization	Local reactions: irritation, itching, rash Systemic effects if serum concentration in toxic range

PABA, para-aminobenzoic acid.

Summary

- Pediatric pain assessment and management requires special consideration.
- Appropriate weight-based dosing is important for adequate pain management.

Suggested Reading

American Academy of Pediatrics. Prevention and management of pain in the neonate: An update. Pediatrics 2006;118(5):2231–2237.

American College of Emergency Physicians. Clinical policy: evidence-based approach to pharmacologic agents used in pediatric sedation and analgesia in the emergency department. Ann Emerg Med 2004;44(4):342–377.

American College of Emergency Physicians. Clinical policy: procedural sedation and analgesia in the emergency department. Ann Emerg Med 2005;(45):177–196.

Lago P, Garetti E, Merazzi D, et al. Guidelines for procedural pain in the newborn. Acta Paediatrica 2009;98:932–939.

Young KD. Pediatric procedural pain. Ann Emerg Med 2005;45(2):160–171.

Zempsky WT. Pharmacologic approaches for reducing venous access pain in children. Pediatrics 2008;122:S140–S153.

Zempsky WT, Cravero JP. Committee on Pediatric Emergency Medicine and Section on Anesthesiology and Pain Medicine. Relief of pain and anxiety in pediatric patients in emergency medical systems. Pediatrics 2004;114:1348–1356.

23 Renal and Biliary Colic

Andrew Worster and Rahim Valani

Renal Colic

- Renal colic occurs when calculi are formed in the renal collecting system.
  - Risk factors include family history, bowel disease, increased sodium or oxalate intake, dietary habits, gout, obesity, immobilization, and low urine output.
  - The urinary tract migration of calculi causes local tissue irritation, bleeding and increased tension to the ureteral wall, and submucosal edema.
  - These factors cause local prostaglandin secretion that, in turn, causes smooth muscle spasm and vasodilatation.
  - The latter that causes diuresis, which again increases the tension to the ureteral wall and renal pelvis. As the stone migrates through the urinary tract, the character and location of the pain may change from muscle spasm-type flank pain to ipsilateral groin and genital discomfort and symptoms of cystitis.
- If the stone is large enough, it will cause partial or complete obstruction of the ureter and, eventually, urinary tract and renal capsule distension (hydronephrosis).
- In the industrialized world, urolithiasis typically affects young, healthy adults.
  - Seventy percent are between 20 and 50 years of age with a peak incidence in males at 30 years and two peaks in women at 35 and 55 years.
  - It also affects 1–2% of the Western pediatric population.
  - White populations > Black irrespective of geographical region.
  - Men > women in White and Asian populations.
  - Women > men in Black and Hispanic populations.
- Diagnosis:
  - Urinalysis may reveal hematuria.
  - Computed tomography (CT) is the imaging of choice.
    - ▶ Advantages of CT include no intravenous contrast, visualization of radiolucent calculi, visualization of pathology outside the urinary tract, and shorter examination time.
  - Ultrasound (US) should be considered as the first choice for imaging test in patients with suspected ureteric colic for whom there is concern over the potentially harmful cumulative long-term effect of radiation.

▶ US has been reported to overestimate stone size and, overall, might not be as accurate as CT although the differences between the two may not be clinically significant.

■ Plain radiographs of the kidneys, ureters, and bladder (KUB) have little value in the diagnosis of acute ureteric colic.

■ Management:

● Most (70%) stones 5 mm or less in diameter and half of those from 5.1 to 10.1 mm can be expected to pass spontaneously.

▶ The length of time from symptom onset to spontaneous stone passage can vary from hours to days and patients may remain symptomatic throughout.

● Extracorporeal shock wave lithotripsy (ESWL) and observation with analgesia with or without adjuvant medications to facilitate stone passage, that is, medical expulsive therapy (MET) are the noninvasive management options for patients with a newly diagnosed ureteral stone smaller than 10 mm diameter.

● Nonsteroidal anti-inflammatory drugs (NSAIDs) such as ketorolac and cyclooxygenase-2 (COX-2) inhibitors, which interfere with prostaglandin synthesis and release can reduce the associated pain of acute ureteric colic by blocking the mechanism of action.

● Opioids have long served as the analgesic of choice by these patients and their attending emergency physicians.

● The combination of opioids and NSAIDs has been found to have an additive analgesic effect greater than either medication alone.

● Calcium channel blockers, alpha-adrenergic blockers, beta-adrenergic blockers, prostaglandin-synthesis inhibitors, glyceryl trinitrate, and steroids have all been used as MET.

● The use of antimuscarinics for the treatment of pain from acute ureteric colic secondary to ureteral smooth muscle spasm might be theoretically sound but has no basis in clinical evidence. There is also no evidence supporting diuretics, high-volume fluid therapy, or antimuscarinic agents.

■ Prolonged duration of symptoms is considered a complication of ureteric colic and, like infection and renal function impairment is an indication for invasive, definitive therapy with ureteroscopy, percutaneous nephrolithotomy, or open surgery.

■ Patients older than 60 years are more likely to suffer infection or be admitted to a hospital.

■ PEARL: Always consider abdominal aortic aneurysm in elderly patients who have symptoms consistent with nephrolithiasis.

Biliary Colic

■ Bile is produced by the hepatocyte cells in the liver and stored in the gallbladder.

■ Contraction of the gallbladder is stimulated with the presence of food through vagal impulses and cholecystokinin.

■ Bile is needed for the digestion of lipids.

■ Gallstones occur when one of the components of bile reaches a supersaturation level that results in precipitation.

- Most patients with gallstones are asymptomatic.
- Types of stones include the following:
  - Cholesterol stones.
    - Is the most common type of gallstone.
  - Pigmented stones (about 20% of cases).
    - Black stones—usually in elderly patients or those with diseases involved with intravascular hemolysis.
    - Brown stones—seen with infection.
- Patients can be symptomatic without stones due to biliary sludge or gallbladder dyskinesia.
- Risk factors for cholesterol gallstones include the following:
  - Increase age
  - Female gender
  - Obesity
  - Pregnancy
  - Rapid weight loss
  - Cystic fibrosis
  - Medications—oral contraceptives, ceftriaxone, estrogens, and total parenteral nutrition.
- Patient presents with varying pain, usually located in the right upper quadrant or epigastrium.
  - Usually post-prandial.
  - Associated nausea and vomiting is common.
  - If patient is febrile, consider acute cholecystitis or cholangitis.
- Investigations:
  - Bloodwork.
    - There are no clinical tests that can identify gallstones or biliary colic.
    - Always check liver transaminases (check for hepatitis), alkaline phosphatase (to determine if there are common bile duct stones), and lipase (for gallstone pancreatitis).
- Radiological investigations.
  - X-ray.
    - Limited utility as only 10–15% of stones have a high concentration of calcium to be seen on plain radiography.
    - The stone must have at least 4% calcium by weight to be radio-opaque.
  - US—has a high specificity (>98%) and sensitivity (>95%), which makes it the imaging of choice.
    - Presence of thickened gallbladder wall (>5 mm), pericholecystic fluid, and positive sonographic Murphy's sign are signs of acute cholecystitis.
  - Oral cholecystography—now replaced by US.
  - CT—useful if suspecting other etiology for patient's pain. Although not an ideal test, it can detect certain gallstones but is superseded by US.

- Magnetic resonance cholangio-pancreatogram—limited utility due to expense and better tests such as US to determine the presence of stones in the gallbladder.
- Useful for looking the hepatic, cystic, and common bile ducts, and choledocholithiasis.
- Management:
  - Fluid and electrolyte correction.
  - Anti-emetic such as Metoclopramide 10 mg IV or Dimenhydrinate 50 mg IV.
  - Anti-spasmodic—Glycopyrrolate 0.2 mg IV push that can be given every 10 minutes up to three doses.
  - Analgesia—Morphine 2–5 mg IV titrated for pain relief.
  - Anti-inflammatory agents—Ketorolac 30 mg IV.
  - Antibiotics are suspected or proven acute cholecystitis.
  - Definitive management is cholecystectomy.
  - Limited utility of oral bile acids.
- Complications of gallstones include the following:
  - Acute cholecystitis
  - Cholangitis
  - Choledocholithiasis
  - Pancreatitis
  - Gallstone ileus
  - Gallbladder empyema
  - Mirizzi syndrome—external compression of the common bile duct. The obstruction is due to gallstone in the cystic duct or Hartmann's pouch.

Suggested Reading

Buckley RG. Cholelithiasis. In: Shaider J, Hayden SR, Wolfe R, Barkin R, Rosen P, eds. Rosen and Barkin's 5 minute emergency medicine consult, 3rd ed. Philadelphia, PA: Lippincott Williams and Wilkins, 2006.

Chari RS, Shah SA. Biliary system. In: Townsend CM, Beauchamp RD, Evers BM, Mattox KL, eds. Sabiston textbook of surgery, 18th ed. St. Louis, MO: WB Saunders, 2008.

Cui H, Kelly JJ. Cholelithiasis. In: Domino F, ed. 5-Minute clinical consult 2011, 19th ed. Philadelphia, PA: Lippincott Williams and Wilkins, 2011.

Guss DA, Oyama LC. Disorders of the liver and biliary tract. In: Marx J, Hockberger R, Walls R, eds. Rosen's emergency medicine: concepts and clinical practice, 7th ed. Philadelphia, PA: Mosby. 2009.

Henderson SO, Swadron S, Newton E. Comparison of intravenous ketorolac and meperidine in the treatment of biliary colic. J Emerg Med 2002;23(3):237–241.

Meyers D, Feldstein DA. Initial treatment of biliary colic: are NSAIDs better than opiates? WMJ 2005;104(4):9, 63.

Olsen JC, McGrath NA, Schwarz DG, et al. A double-blind randomized clinical trial evaluating the analgesic efficacy of ketorolac versus butorphanol for patients with suspected biliary colic in the emergency department. Acad Emerg Med 2008;15(8):718–722.

Pietrow PK, Karellas ME. Medical management of common urinary calculi. Am Fam Physician 2006;74(1):86–94.

Rosenstein D, McAninch JW. Urologic emergencies. Med Clin North Am 2004;88: 495–518.

Singh A, Alter H, Littlepage A. A systematic review of medical therapy to facilitate passage of ureteral calculi. Ann Emerg Med 2007;50:552–563.

Teichman JM. Clinical practice. Acute renal colic from ureteral calculus. N Engl J Med 2004;350(7):684–693.

Worster A, Richards C. Fluids and diuretics for acute ureteric colic. Cochrane Database Syst Rev 2005;(3):CD004926.

Index